Ancient Indian Massage

Traditional Massage Techniques
Based on the Ayurveda

HARISH JOHARI

Munshiram Manoharlal
Publishers Pvt. Ltd.

ISBN 81-215-0008-7
This edition 2000
© 1984 **Johari**, Pratibha

Printed and published by
Munshiram Manoharlal Publishers Pvt. Ltd.,
Post Box 5715, 54 Rani Jhansi Road,
New Delhi 110 055.

Ancient
Indian Massage

Other books by the author :
Dhanwantri *(English and Spanish)*

Leela : The Game of Self-Knowledge
   (English, Dutch, German, Spanish and Greece)

The Chakra Colouring Book *(English, German)*

Tratak, Meditation on Light

Contents

Preface

s food is a necessity for the organism from birth to death, so is massage to the human organism. Food provides nourishment from external sources to the organism, whereas massage excites the internal resources and provides nourishment in the form of proteins, glucose, and other vitalizing chemicals which are within the system. Massage, like a mother, preserves the body energy and saves the organism from decay. It also works as a cleanser and helps the organism in discharging toxins out of the body through sweat, urine and mucous; thus rejuvenating the body.

Massage is the first friend which serves the human organism from the time of birth. In India it is a tradition to massage the body from the first day, which continues to at least the third year every day. After three years of age the routine changes and massage is done at least once or twice a week, up to about the sixth year. Afterwards, the child is able to massage others and get massage in return. This continues until he starts playing and doing physical exercises.

Weekly massage is a family scene, everyone does it. With the advance of age when a child attains the state of youth, he/she gets interested in building the body. The next stage comes when one gets married and receives the massage from his/her partner (the wife gives her husband massage every day till the end of her life). In old age there are grandchildren to play with and give massage to the grandparents. Thus, for the majority, massage is a part of life.

There are also ceremonial massages. The one which is compulsory is massage before marriage, which provides the glaze and the look of a bride/bridegroom to the young couple. This massage is done with chemicals and oils. Massage before marriage relaxes the one being married, gives stamina, provides psychic strength and increases beauty. Another compulsory massage is to a lady after the delivery of a child. This massage is done daily for minimum 40 days.

In ancient days, life was simple and close to nature. Modern age is the age of greed and competition. Life has become strenuous. There is stress on the nerves every moment. In this modern age of stress and strain massage is a must. The speed of everything has increased and there are unnatural shocks shaking the nervous system every moment. The literature now available on massage shows an inner urge in people in the western world to find natural methods of relaxing and vitalizing the human organism. Massage is the most natural and powerful method of relaxing and at the same time rejuvenating the body.

It is now becoming known to many people that this modern way of living is not right, yet it is impossible to go back to Nature and start living once again in the way our ancestors lived five hundred years ago. We shall have to avoid the use of drugs and chemicals in order to keep our body chemistry in good shape. Some chemicals used as preservatives have become part of our food industry. We can not avoid these if we do not discard packaged food, milk and cheese — which is almost impossible if we live in this era. So there remains only one alternative — to learn and practise such devices which would help the system flush out these toxins as regularly as they are ingested. The skin also plays a very important role in excreting waste materials and toxins.

Massage is one of the few well known remedies for helping all such problems. The use of natural, organic foods; water; earth; sunlight and air (along with massage) can prove a fantastic remedy.

Massage works on the body on both levels:
1. Physical
2. Psyche

1. Physical:

Rubbing of the body produces heat and increases blood circulation, it affects the lymphatic system and supplies more nourishment to the blood.

2. Psyche:

Through touch, massage works on the nervous system and affects the circulation of growth hormones. *All feelings and fantasies of the massager are transmitted to the person getting the massage.*

As a child massage was given to me everyday but I do not remember myself as a small baby. When I recall my childhood I find myself massaging the holy feet of my mother sometimes - and most of the time I see myself giving massage to my Grandfather, who was also at the same time giving his precious instructions to me on the subject how to massage. This was just a play, so far as I remember I learnt how to massage properly in 1949 and later on in 1952-53 it became a part of my daily routine when I joined the wrestling ground (Akhara) at Jaunpur, which was situated right in front of my house. Massage was essential for all who came to the wrestling ground.

Shri Jaswanta Singh Mukhtar (Advocate) - our landlord - was very interested in wrestling - and massage and he appointed Pabbar Pahalwan (Wrestler) to come and instruct me in wrestling and massage. Ustad Pabbar Pahalwan was a wrestler of provincial fame specially very popular in Eastern Uttar Pradesh, because of his engagements he could not come regularly to teach me - and most of my training was done under Shri Jaswanta Singh himself besides Shri Bhrigu Nath and Bodhan - famous wrestlers of Jaunpur. To massage the teachers and to get massaged by them was very healthy; it increased my stamina, vigour, vitality and inner strength, gave me self control, strong will-power and endurance, which later helped me in my work as a sculptor.

In 1957-58 while I was living at Rampur I had the fortune of meeting the most handsome and wise wrestler Siddique Khan, son of the famous royal wrestler of Rampur Sohrab Khan, who was also a healer. Siddique Bhai agreed to instruct me in wrestling and in art of massage. Siddique Khan brought my attention to the MARMAS (vital points) and explained to me secrets of rubbing, kneading and squeezing.

My understanding about massage was further enriched by my Ayurvedic medicine man friend and teacher Shri Rameshwar Prasad Pande. He prescribed massage to his patients very frequently and was able to achieve quick recovery with a combined effect of medicine, diet and massage. It was here in his enlightened company I learnt about the three humours Wind, Bile and Mucous.

Oil massage and massage of pressure points made a deep impression on my mind - and when I came to the Western Hemisphere I was astonished to see that very few persons here massaged with oil. Massage is very essential for people living in cold climate. Cold climate, lack of exercises and more intellectual work - all combined together create dryness and poor circulation of blood in the body and massage is the only remedy which could help a healthy and wholesome growth of body and mind.

I thank my teachers and students, who helped me in making the present book on massage, which can provide some practical help to people interested in physical and mental. well-being.

I thank my student Dan Conrod for making the primary drawings of massage book which later on I improved - and made them suitable for the book.

HARISH JOHARI

363, PANJABPURA
BAREILLY - U.P. INDIA.

Introduction

Ancient Indian Massage: The Lymphatic Massage
A Preventive Health Technique

Michael L. Gerber, M.D.

Treating balance in one's own body depends upon proper nutrition, adequate sleep and proper exercise. Working with these areas of body maintenance will help to assure a long and productive life. With the passage of time, however, balancing these factors becomes increasingly difficult. Exercise, for example, frequently becomes inadequate with advancing age bringing about a number of serious emotional and physical problems.

Each of these areas of bodily maintenance has fascinated scientists and physicians throughout history and around the world. Ancient Greek and Roman physicians thought about the body in terms of keeping it in balance by manipulating these pillars of good health. The Eastern medicine of the Hindus and Chinese of today is likewise concerned with balance.

The Hindus, for example, use techniques preserved in the Sanskrit texts as old as 2,500 year—back at least 2,500 years which deal with this art of maintaining balance in the body. This system is called the Ayurveda, literally translated as the science of longevity. Ayurveda, like the Chinese Acupuncture system, is principally concerned with the individual's balance in diet and everyday living habits so that he stays free of physical and emotional diseases. These Indian doctors give a different diet for each person that changes with the seasons of the year and even with the days of the week.

Both systems also work by adjusting the intercellular fluid in the body the organic, which we call lymph, in order to create an electrical and chemical balance among organ systems to preserve their proper functioning. Acupuncturists use needles, local skin heating and massage to effect this probable balancing of the DC currents in the lymph where as the Hindus use, oil massage of the foot or hand to accomplish many of the same things.

As with all knowledge, this concern for balancing has recycled to catch the attention of modern scientists. And, like many rediscovered ancient ideas, these concepts of health seem to agree, in some areas, with modern medical research data from the West. This linkage of ancient and modern may provide new techniques to be used in the practice of one's personal routine of preventive health care. As everyman becomes more able to deal with his own body balance, he will not only have less disease but he will also be physically and emotionally stronger and a great deal happier.

The concept of preventive medicine is new in the United States but will undoubtedly find a place in our culture. We are reaching a point where we are becoming increasingly more conscious of our bodies and the need to keep them in the best possible condition. Staying in the best condition reflects in all our life's activities—both for work and play. Daily balancing of our physical vehicle provides not only maximum performance with optimum wear but also a richer emotional life.

One topic of current interest in our investigations of new and ancient techniques for balancing is the Lymphatic massage. We will examine its importance for Westerners, especially for gerontology, and look at the interesting scientific correlations of this technique. The Lymphatic massage has rather striking effects, especially relaxation of the subject, which makes it a likely candidate to be used as a therapeutic tool in the West.

A look at the lymphatic system from the point of view of the East and West is very interesting. This system has received very little attention by Western scientists until recent years primarily because of its delicate nature and the ease with which these vessels can be overlooked or disrupted on gross disection of the body. This system which is quite necessary for our survival has been studied recently in connection with cancer research by more refined microscopic and staining techniques which enable scientists to better understand lymph flow as well as lymph constituents.

Although a comprehensive review of lymph is beyond the scope of this book, we will attempt to provide a few basic facts about the lymphatic system. Lymph is found everywhere outside the cells in the human body with the exceptions of the brain, bone marrow and deep inside skeletal muscle. It is a clear or milky coloured fluid which originates by leakage from blood capillaries. This system carries nutrients to the cells and waste products and foreign particles away from the cells, it then passes into small lymph vessels. These delicate lymph vessels can distend up to six times larger than the accompanying vein but are usually only slightly larger. These lymph vessels travel a short distance and then enter a lymph node. Here if there are any bacteria, viruses, foreign particles or cellular debris in the lymph they will be eaten by large cells in the lymph node and be destroyed. Another lymph vessel takes out the freshly cleaned lymph from the other side of the lymph node and moves it on to the heart. Lymph vessels have valves so that the fluid flows in only one direction—towards the heart. The lymph flow finally rejoins the blood stream at the base of the neck where the largest lymphatic collecting vessel, called the thoracic duct, empties its lymph into the internal jugular vein and there it mixes with the blood.

Lymph has many elements which make it important for the body maintenance. It contains roughly half the concentration of protein one finds in blood plasma. Since lymph flows back into the blood stream at a rate of one to six quarts per day, depending upon the amount of exercise, it is equivalent to giving six units of blood plasma intraveinously per day. This system returns the serum proteins to the blood which escape normally into the lymphatic space. This is very large amount of protein every day. The body literally feeds itself with its own preprocessed food or lymph. It seems reasonable that a great diminution of this protein rich fluid would alter the body's metabolism.

As it has been widely evidenced that the rate of lymph flow depends upon several variables. For example, a subject who is lying in bed in poor physical condition may have as little as one quart of lymph recirculated into the blood stream daily whereas an active ambulatory subject can have as much as six quarts of lymph returned to his circulation in a day. It is interesting that lymph, for the most part, depends on muscular contraction to make it flow back toward the heart. Lymph from arms, legs and head does not move measurably while at rest. It is very frequently mentioned by experimenters in this field that as a part of their routine of collection of lymph samples it is necessary to massage the area of interest to get the lymph to flow at all. Massage greatly increases lymph flow. In one experiment, lymph flow was measured in the hind leg of a dog. At rest no lymph flowed, but by rhythmically squeezing the paw of that leg pressure increased in the lymph vessel from 0 to 50 centimeters of water.

Among the many important aspects of lymph physiology, we might mention that lymph contains a great number of lymphocytes which are the white blood cells (w b c) responsible for maintaining the body's circulating immunological resistance. A large portion of these infection fighting cells are formed in the lymph nodes. The thoracic duct output of these white blood cells in man per day is equal to the total amount of these cells in the blood, in the rat it is twenty-seven times as great.

By and large the composition of lymph is similar to that of blood plasma. There are, however, some exceptions which may prove to be of interest. Lymph contains a significant amount of the essential amino acid tryptophan when compared with dietary intake and blood levels of this relatively scare but important compound. Tryptophan is necessary for serotonin and melatonin formation which are important body substances necessary for energy production and nervous and hormonal balance. Lymph contains high levels of all other amino acids, proteins (especially rich in albumin) and most body enzymes. Of interest among these enzymes are high levels of dopamine beta hydroxylase (implicated in the pathogenesis of schizophrenia) and histaminase, the enzyme which breaks down histamine. When histamine levels in the body become elevated it can cause high gastric acidity, lethargy, itching, headaches, painful muscles and painful lymph nodes. Histamine is also the major chemical involved in the body's allergic response. These allergic phenomena, such as hay fever, manifest by symptoms of swelling and inflammation of the nasal mucous membranes, nasal obstruction, reddening of the eyes, itching and cough. Indeed, one might speculate that lymph, which has thirty times as much histaminase as blood, could be the body's own natural anti-histamine.

There are many other interesting correlations which link one's state of health with one's state of lymphatic functioning. At this point however, let us look at the Eastern medicine approach, especially Lymphatic Massage and see how they view this system.

The Indian Ayurvedic system of medicine calls the lymph system the Kapha or mucous carrying system. This tradition developed a massage that includes pressure points (they correspond remarkably with the anatomical position of lymph nodes) which are gently massaged with organic oils (principally mustard seed oil, coconut oil, and almond oil) to achieve a balance in the body's energy system. Kapha has been interpreted by modern Vedyas (Ayurvedic doctors) as being a property of lymph. Increasing the Kapha activity is purported to increase the nourishment of the body and give proper articulation of joints, fortitude, patience, solidarity, sexual stamina and abstinence. Most frequently this massage is performed by massaging only the feet, the hands, or the head of the recipient. Through regular massage, they feel that the balance is restored to the body's electro-chemical pathways and serves as a preventive health technique. In the Hindu culture this massage is generally performed within the family or extended family with children massaging the grandparents in the household and husband and wife exchanging massage. Youthful energy is thus circulated throughout the household. The subjective effects include rapid relaxation that frequently results in light sleep. It is also useful to relieve pain of skeletal muscle origin and may find utility in elevating mood. Some of our patients who have received this massage describe feelings of peacefulness and diminished anxiety. If this observation holds true, it could be a valuable new tool to produce mental relaxation by a simple physical technique.

In Acupuncture, at least part of the effect is derived from stimulation of lymph. In fact, a map of the Acupuncture points corresponds quite well to a chart of the body's lymph nodes. Acupuncturists feel that they are dealing with the electrical currents present in the body and that by manipulation of the intercellular fluid or lymph with needles, moxybustion (heating) or massage these electrical fields can be balanced. They also recommend balancing at regular intervals to prevent the onset of disease which results from imbalance in this system.

The implications of these approaches to preventive medicine and body balancing could be extremely important for the Western patient. This massage technique also provides an avenue to make new physical contact between the young and the old. For example, students and volunteers could easily learn and use this massage with geriatrics patients on hospital in-patient services and for senior citizens in general.

SUMMARY

Balancing the functions of the body is becoming of greater interest in the West as we learn techniques to accomplish this task. Acupuncturists use needles to balance body energies while Ayurvedic physicians use oil massage as their tool for physical balance. Both systems define good health care as essentially preventive in nature.

It is becoming increasingly suggestive that the little studied lymphatic system of the body plays a role in this balancing process which may involve chemical pathways already known and studied by Western scientists as well as through electrical currents previously unknown in the West.

The Lymphatic massage may be particularly useful when employed in a preventive health care system for the layman, especially the elderly whose lymphatic system is already compromised due to regression of lymph tissue with increasing age, diminished daily exercise and reduced efficiency of the heart.

Lymphatic massage causes a number of subjective changes in mood which are generally relaxing in nature but need to be experienced to be appreciated. This technique may find acceptance by Americans more readily than pain creating balancing manoeuvre The Lymphatic massage is painless, actually quite pleasant, and can be easily performed by the lay public or professional therapists.

4

Implications of Research

Lymphatic massage is an Indian massage technique, several thousand years old, which uses natural oils (mainly mustard seed oil and almond oil). It is a precise, gentle massage which focuses on the body's lymphatic pathways. The effects of lymphatic massage are striking. These positive results have prompted the TRI (TANTRA RESEARCH INSTITUTE) Medical Research Staff to engage in research to elucidate the mechanism of the body's physiological response to this massage and the implications for its use as a therapeutic tool for clinicians.

The massage technique is pointed towards increasing lymph flow (in the skin) as well as lymph movement in the larger lymphatic vessels and lymph nodes of the body. The hands gently stimulate lymphatic flow and avoid creating pain of resistance. Most people find themselves nearly asleep following their first foot massage or in a light trance, enjoying a sense of relief and calm. Many have found interesting sensations of currents of energy flowing throughout the body.

In this introduction we will review the physiology of the body's lymph system and some experimental findings associated with the lymphatic system. Some historical notes on massage and a few of its practical applications are also included.

Massage has an interesting history and takes its roots back at least 2,400 years in India. Lymphatic massage, associated with Marmas (vital points) tradition, has been carried forward in its most developed form into modern times by wrestlers in India. These men are most concerned with keeping their bodies in excellent condition. The best type of energy exchange is considered through men to men and women to woman massage.

The ancient Indians felt that the benefits of massage were mediated by increasing the flow of lymph in lymph vessels and ascribed to lymph the properties of increasing viscosity, nourishment, solidarity, sexual stamina, good articulation of joints, fortitude, patience and abstinence.

In the West, oil massage (anointing with oil) has been known since biblical times and was prescribed by Hippocrates, Galen, Pare, and most famous doctors in Western medical history. They felt it exerted a favourable influence on the course of disease.

Western medical men have also been aware of the lymphatic system. These vessels carrying 'white blood' were known to Hippocrates (406-377BC), and the 'chuliferous vessels' were described at length by Herophilus (300 BC). This system was rediscovered 1800 years later by Andreas Vesalius of Brussels (1514-1564) and Bartolomeous Eustachius of Rome (1520-1574), both believing it to be a part of the venous system. Olaus Rudbeck (1630-1708) discovered that lymphatic vessels had valves permitting one way flow of lymph, and that it was a separate fluid returning system in the body.

In modern times, medical anatomists and surgeons have used a variety of staining and die techniques to discover the exact route of the lymph movement as it returns from each organ and extremity of the body to the heart.

X-ray localisation (lymphangiograms) shows the exact location of lymph vessels and nodes. Amazingly enough, there is exact anatomical correlatiom between pressure points/marmas and massage movements of the ancient Hindu system and lymph nodes and vessels as shown by modern scientific technique.

What is lymph? Lymph is the fluid which normally leaks out of blood capillaries throughout the body and contains most of the same elements as blood plasma, proteins amino acids, glucose, fats, hormones, enzymes, salts, and lymphocytes (white blood cells which fight infection). The lymphatic system is responsible for returning protein lost naturally to the tissues and extracellular spaces back to the blood stream. In quantity, lymph contains about half as much protein as can be found in blood plasma with each region and organ of the body returning its own unique lymph composition. For example, fat soluble vitamins A, D, E, and K are absorbed by intestinal lymph vessels called lacteals, which remove fat from the intestines during digestion. Kidney lymph is high in histaminase, liver lymph is high in proteins and enzymes, etc. Lymph also aids circulation by maintaining the balance of the fluids in the body. Edema or swelling of the body is due, in part, to inadequate lymph return.

The paramount importance of lymph is that it provides cellular components for the body's immune response. It contains lymphocytes and plasma cells (both white blood cells), and phagocytic reticuloendothelial cells which destroy foreign matter, bacteria and alien cells which invade the body. Lymphocytes (made in part by lymph nodes) provide the body with circulating immunological resistance. In man, the daily output of lymphocytes from the thoracic duct (largest lymph channel) has been found to equal the number of lymphocytes in the blood.

All lymph moves from the peripheral parts of the body (arms, legs, head) through lymph vessels which are usually closely associated with veins and arteries and empty into the thoracic duct which lies along the midline of the trunk between the aorta and spinal column. The thoracic duct then returns lymph to the large veins near the base of the neck. Once into these large veins above the heart, the lymph fluid mixes with the blood and is pumped throughout the body by the heart. The thoracic duct delivers between two to six liters of lymph back to the blood stream daily in man, dependent on his activity. Thoracic duct lymph flow is aided by valves in the lymph vessels, aortic pulsations, respiration (deep breath), increasing peripheral lymph flow (as in massage and exercise), increased output of kidney lymph (which accompanies diuresis; i.e. increasing urine output), and increased abdominal pressure. General measures to increase lymph flow include exercise, anozia (holding the breath), standing on the head (gravity), and increasing local skin temperature.

Once we have increased lymph flow by lymphatic massage, what are the theoretical mechanisms causing its mental and physical effects? There are several likely processes which may be involved. First, lymph possesses a relatively large amount of the amino acid tryptophan, especially when compared with the dietary intake. It likewise has a large amount of albumin (protein), glucose and histaminase (breaks down histamine). Hypothetically, blood amino acids like tryptophan increase after massage. An increase in plasma tryptophan subsequently causes a parallel increase in the neuro-transmitter (chemical between nerve endings), and serotonin, which is made from tryptophan. Serotonin has been implicated in several psychiatric diseases with low levels of its metablite found by researchers in depression and schizophrenia.

All the functions of serotonin have yet to be elucidated, but depletion of serotonin from the brain by parachlorophenylalanine (PCPA) (a serotonin inhibitor) has been shown by numerous investigators to cause irritability, aggressiveness, abnormal fear reactions, tremor, incessant grooming and apparent hallucinatory behaviour in dogs, cats and monkeys. In man the relatively few studies available describe similar mental effects such as depression, florid hallucinations, paranoia, severe headache, anxiety and irritability after giving PCPA. So, as serotonin is depleted (decreased) this assortment of responses may be expected. Giving albumin (protein) bound tryptophan to the brain through proper diet and lymphatic massage should, theoretically, increase brain serotonin. In practice lymphatic massage seems to relieve symptoms like those caused by serotonin depletion, anxiety, irritability, etc. This may well be one link in the process.

Melatonin, a newly discovered brain hormone whose parent compound is serotonin, is also synthesised from tryptophan (tryptophan forms serotonin which, in turn, forms melatonin). Melatonin is rhythmically secreted in the pineal gland of the brain. Radioactive tryptophan has been found to accumulate in pineal, so we can assume the pineal uses it to form serotonin and melatonin. The pineal gland has a diurnal rhythm and is sensitive to light. During the day the pineal produces high levels of serotonin, and at night produces high levels of melatonin.

Melatonin has been found to decrease thyroid activity, adrenal and gonadal activity as well as diminish growth hormone and melanocyte stimulating hormone levels. In all, melatonin decreases protein synthesis in the hypothalmus and pituitary, resulting in a decrease in six of the seven anterior pituitary hormones (three of six confirmed in man). Melatonin turns down the body's hormonal activity. Giving melatonin to human results in sleep or sedation (depending upon the dose and way of administration), vivid dreams, EEG changes which resemble those of a meditative state, and a feeling of well being and moderate elation.

Melatonin, like serotonin, is made from tryptophan and may be another neuro-chemical means which causes the pleasant, calming effects one experiences during lymphatic massage.

Lymph has several other chemical differences from blood plasma which may be involved in mediating the body's response to lymphatic massage. Many researchers have noted that lymph contains approximately thirty times as much histaminase as in blood. Histaminase is a diamine oxidase, an enzyme, which breaks down diamines such as histamine and is found most concentrated in lymph, kidneys, and intestines. We know that increases of histamine are associated with many pathological body processes in man and cause headache, marked increase in stomach acidity and lethargy. Histamine is also found in abnormally high quantities in enlarged, painful lymph nodes. Empirically, we have noted that lymphatic massage relieves sore muscles. Perhaps it is the local movement of lymph (high in histaminase) through these enlarged tissues by lymphatic massage that causes improvement in painful, swollen tissue areas (high in histamine). Also of interest is the cutaneous skin response in these painful areas. When one presses firmly on these tender areas a red mark similar in appearance to the classical histamine flare appears on the surrounding skin, as if one had injected histamine into that area.

Diminishing histamine may also have important central effects such as diminishing gastric acidity (stimulating stomach acid secretion by administering histamine is the classical test of stomach acid production), improving headache, decreasing the allergic response (mediated by histamine) to environmental allergies (hay fever, etc.). If lymph does have a natural anti-histamine function, it may prove to be one important mediator of the effects of lymphatic massage.

Another interesting set of studies in animals show changes in brain structure and activity if lymph drainage of the brain is cut off. After ligating (tying off) all the lymph vessels in the necks of dogs, researchers noted the following: the dogs' brains became edematous (swollen), cells in important brain areas became disrupted, there was an increased intracranial pressure (sign of abnormality), they had a diminished seizure threshold (convulsions occur more easily), they showed EEG (brain wave) abnormalities and exhibited dullness and decreased reactivity to stimuli.

In men and women stiff-neck muscles and swollen lymph nodes (often resembling a small string of pearls down the sides of the neck) have been noted in patients suffering from schizophrenia and other nervous disorders in the absence of demonstrable infection in the nasopharyngeal passages. Since swollen nodes indicate a diminished lymph flow, in this case from the head, it is tempting to speculate that some degree of lymph stasis (non-movement) is involved in these psychiatric disorders.

These research issues have been raised so the reader might have an idea of the type of inquiry being pursued by the TRI Medical Research staff. The story of lymph and its connection with hormones, amino acids, neurotransmitters, scrotonin, melatonin, histamine, etc., is slowly unfolding. We feel that with proper research emphasis, meaningful scientific links will be established between lymphatic massage, diet, daily habits and body chemistry which will improve our quality of living and give clinicians valuable new tools for therapy.

Thus far we have touched on some of the scientific connections of lymphatic massage. Of greater importance at this stage of our knowledge is the historical and practical information about this massage.

The effects of the massage vary with the time of day. During the day, it relaxes and refreshed, giving increased energy. In the evening it is more tranquilizing.

The massage has many uses. We have found it excellent for relieving headaches, muscle aches, anxiety, weakness, irritability, feelings of insecurity and agitation, and it is a *powerful,* non-drug method to promote sleep. Our medical staff has found it useful for calming psychotic individuals as well as giving rest and improved mood to depressed patients. Likewise, those persons withdrawing from drugs, alcohol, heroin, amphetamines and LSD have shown good response to lymphatic massage.

While briefly mentioning its uses we must include the hospitalised and elderly patients who have enjoyed this massage. In this group of people, normal lymph flow is impeded by lack of exercise, poor breathing habits and diminished capabilities of their circulatory system. We have found, in the bed-ridden, chronic anger, insomnia, fearfulness, body aches and pains are ameliorated by lymphatic massage. It is an excellent way to establish rapport with the elderly. We feel lymphatic massage is an especially good means of transferring energy from the youth (high school and college students) to the elderly.

At the opposite end of the age spectrum, children seem to respond very well to lymphatic massage especially when agitated, irritable, overly tired, unable to sleep of simply in need of touching. Little ones love lymphatic massage and parents find that spending a few minutes in massaging their children soon replaces less loving and less efficient methods of inducing change.

For man and wife these massage techniques offer a variety of new experiences plus tangible method of energy transfer. We have found that the head massage, for example, produces mental alertness, diminished anger and irritability and greatly improves one's mood. These effects are most pronounced in the morning.

From the Indian historical background and from our own experience, we have noted that foot massage is effective for increasing the male's sexual endurance before ejaculation and is good for both partners so that they synchronize with each others temperature, pulse and breath rate before lovemaking. Lymphatic massage also encourages a diminished speed of the sexual experience allowing more subtle energies to be appreciated.

Of the greatest import is that lymphatic massage increases one's *self awareness*. For lack of a better description many people experience what they call 'energy flows' during lymphatic massage which seem to travel from one point in the body to another and cause an inward focusing of attention. The appreciation of this kind of subtle energy is useful in regulating one's daily habits, diet, and meditation. Some practices bring this energy flow downward toward the anus; others bring it up toward the head. Balancing one's body chemistry and nervous activity is aided by working with these subtle feelings.

Lymphatic massage has had a significant impact on those who have learned it—doctors, psychologists, lawyers, firemen, policemen, students, housewives and businessmen. All have found this massage to be powerful, gentle and practical whether in a clinical setting or at home. We have found that Americans are coming to realize that the responsibility for maintaining good health rests with the individual and his daily habits. We feel lymphatic massage can increase one's body knowledge and serve as a tool to maintain good health and introduce practices necessary to attain supra normal health.

I
Principles of Massage

One who follows the natural contours and flows of the body insures the most effective massage.

One who works counter to the natural formation of the body creates imbalance and disease.

Intricacies of Massage

To be a good massager, one needs to look at the formation and function of the musculature. One who follows the natural contours and flows of the body insures the most effective massage. One who works counter to the natural formation of the body creates imbalance and disease.

The body can be divided into three general regions:

- The region from the base of the spine to the head (torso and head).

- The region from the pelvis to the toes.

- The region from the collar-bones to the fingertips.

The shape of the muscles in the first region—from skullcap to tailbone—is round and the energy flows from up to down and vice versa. In the formation of the limbs in an embryo, this part develops first and as a unit. The head develops first, then the rest of the fertilized ovum undergoing mitosis and meosis becomes the rest of the torso, up to the base of the spine. Thus we see that these parts are actually a unit and should be massaged as a unit.

In the second region, energy moves down from the pelvis to the feet as the body pushes against the earth and the force of gravity with the legs. The circulation is downward as this part keeps in contact with the earth and it is the lower region of the body. This is the part of the body designed for the function of pushing. In *Shakti-Pat Maha Yoga* (transference of energy) the feet of the *Guru* are supposed to be worshipped because it is through the feet that the *Guru* transfers his energy to the disciple in order to open knots and make the flow of energy free in the spine and to promote spiritual growth. It is said that *Swami Rama Krishna Paramhamsa* transferred his energy into *Swami Vivekananda* by hitting him through his feet.

In the third region, the upper arms, elbows, forearms, wrists, palms and fingers form a co-ordinated whole to draw energy into the body. This is the pulling section. In both the second and third regions the formation of the musculature is linear, and the energy flows from the torso downwards and outwards.

The hands are used to draw energy into the body
   to pull
   to express emotions
   to help the psyche to express
   and to save man.

Thus these hands work as a vehicle of *prana* (vital life breath). In dance, hands make *mudras* (postures) to tell the audience the feelings and the story. In worship they serve as connectors, they raise the energy level and help psychic currents to flow. The fingertips are the most important part of hands, because they transmit energy. All fine jobs a man does are done by fingers. Fingers are used in different ways by all workers and fine artists alike. There are many miracles related to the sensation of touching, the transference of energy through the fingertips from one man to another (or God to man, as Michaelangelo depicted on the ceiling of the Sistine Chapel). Fingertips point the way.

According to the structuring of each of these three major divisions the oil must be so applied. While working on the front part of the torso the hands should move downwards from face to neck, to chest, to abdomen, to waist. On the back side, however, the hands should move upwards from the base of the spine to the base of the skull, and outwards from the area of the ribcage.

If massage of the back portion of the torso is begun at the neck and moved downwards along the spine to the pelvis, energy is drawn down with the hands. Most sensual games begin in this manner, with patting of the rear of the skull and hands gradually moving downwards. *This flow of energy works counter to the principles of massage for better flow of energy upwards and should not be used except for sex play.*

II
Sequence of Massage

Massage adopted as a daily practise offers much pleasurable benefit. Body heat and vitality increase as the heart and the circulatory system open up to provide fresh oxygen and vital energy to all parts of the body while simultaneously flushing out waste gases and toxins.

It should be remembered that for the maximum benefit from massage the massaging should commence from the upper leg—outside; then the inside of the upper leg should be massaged. Outside is male and inside female. After this, lower legs should be massaged and then the foot massage should be given, following the same outside and inside principle. After this, hips and sides should be worked with, and the lower back should be massaged—moving upwards—covering the upper back. Then the front massage should be performed. After this, arms should be massaged. The head should always be massaged last.

Properly executed, however, massage helps the body to become light, active and energetic. Regular massage, even once a week, prevents development of most skin disorders including:

eczema,
blisters,
scabies and
seborrhea.

It also increases intelligence, ready wit, stamina, sexual vitality (semen), self confidence and beauty. Massage is therapeutically used for:

neurasthenia,
headaches,
insomnia,
gout,
polio,
fatness,
obesity
and mental disorders.

It balances the three *doshas* . . . wind, bile and mucous.

III
Importance of the Spine
in Massage

Human Spine—seat of miracles

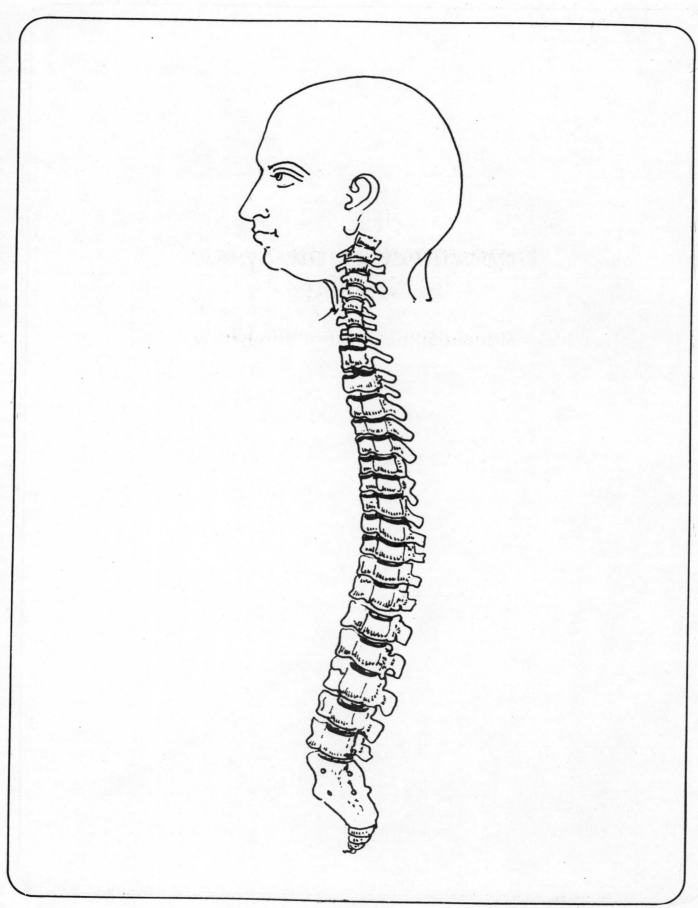

I n dealing with the human organism we have to understand the importance of the spine. The human spine is the seat of miracles. *Yoga* and *Tantra,* the sciences which deal with evolution of human consciousness, are full of the description of the mysterious powers of *Kundalini,* the serpent power, which operates through the spine. The spine is the seat of all *chakras,* psychic centers, except the sixth *chakra* and beyond. The central nervous system as well as the autonomous nervous system also work through the spine. The sympathetic and para-sympathetic nervous-systems also operate through the spine. All healers in the past, and those who work with natural methods of healing in the present times, accept the importance of the spine and work on the spine in their own way. For a massager, the spine is the base of the youth and glamour. If the spine is properly aligned and strong, the vital life force will flow in the body for longer duration. If the spine is in the right shape, a man will think right, act right, and live an energetic life. One who is learning about massage must learn how to put all the vertebrae in proper alignment. Another important thing to remember is the role of the spinal fluid in maintaining health, vigour, vitality and virility. He should understand that massage of the spine alone can cure weak nerves and all psychic disorders.

We have mentioned that the spine is the seat of psychic centers. The psychic centers work through the ductless glands and influence the body chemistry which is registered as emotional changes by the human brain. By massaging the spine the massager can slowly bring about a change in body chemistry and release one from all tensions.

The spine is made up of vertebrae, and through these vertebrae the central nervous system operates, sending its offshoots to the whole body. If we take the body to be an inverted tree, the brain becomes the roots and the spine the trunk. This trunk is the supporter of branches, leaves and fruits. The trunk of the tree upholds the tree against gravitational force, as does the spine. If one sits with his spine erect he is least affected by gravitational force. In all mental and physical disorders the shape of the spine becomes defective and the patient is unable to uphold his spine for any length of time. Mostly, people are not conscious of the shape of the spine, they use backrests and never sit on their own spine. The spine is shaped like a rattle snake. Its shape can be seen in its best form in a walking child . . . a child who has learned running and jumping. Children between the ages of three and six years of age have spines the shape of a snake. This can be seen even up to eighty years of age in some cases, but usually it starts getting deformed after forty-five years of age with the loss of agility and quick response to maturity and ageing.

In diagrams showing back massage, each vertebrae is explained. Here we shall only discuss the shape of the spine, this being one of the most important factors in physical and mental health. It can be clearly observed that in moments of sadness and pessimism the spine becomes loose and does not remain erect. And, in moments of alertness, inspiration and joy the spine becomes erect. The right shape of the spine is directly related to the circulation of vital life fluid in the spine. This vital life fluid is responsible for both physical and mental health. All physical exercises help this circulation and thus all those persons who do exercises regularly feel more inspired and fresh. Twisting of the spine to the right and to the left is a very effective method of putting the spine in the right shape and it is good for increasing the circulation of the spinal fluid. The main work of a massager is to massage the spine not very roughly, and also not very gently. Bearable pressure should be applied on both sides. The massage should be done with the thumbs (as shown in the illustration on back massage)* sometimes fingertips and wrists may also be used, but the thumbs work best for giving continuous massage.

Massage without oil and without pressure is not effective on the spine. The pressure applied should not be unbearable, otherwise the spine will have to exert pressure to counter-balance the external pressure, and this would affect the nerves and brain. Also, the massage should start from the root of the spine and should move upwards. The middle part of the spine should be aligned with a little pressure and the massage should be given on both sides of the spine, with both the thumbs. At the end of each vertebrae, a circular movement should be made, allowing enough time to each vertebrae so that each, in turn, becomes vibrant and alive. If massage is done patiently about 5 grams of oil will be easily absorbed. Then, up to the end of one's life, one will never have any stiffness in his back, no disorder in his kidneys, liver, stomach, lungs or brain. The entire nervous system is dependent upon the spine. Working with the spine is working with the mysterious energy force in the body.

IV
Massage

- *As a daily practise*
- *And exercise*
- *For relaxation*

Massage adopted as a daily practise ensures proper circulation and relaxes muscles, it also removes all tensions and increases the circulation of lymph fluid which provides more oxygen, glucose, proteins, and other vitalising chemicals for the blood which then is circulated in the entire organism.

Massage as a Daily Practice

Those who are desirous of a healthy body, throughout life, should adopt massage as a daily practise. They should massage their body daily for at least thirty to forty-five minutes before bathing. The bath should not be taken immediately after massage. During massage the body becomes hot and the circulation of blood increases. The pores of the body open and, without proper equalisation of temperature, a bath is injurious. Massage adopted as a daily practise ensures proper circulation and relaxes muscles; it also removes all tensions and increases the circulation of lymph fluid which provides more oxygen, glucose, proteins and other vitalising chemicals for the blood which then is circulated in the entire organism.

For those who are young and energetic and interested in building the body, massage is a must. In India and Greece body-builders and wrestlers massage the body daily. The strain taken by muscles in exercises and wrestling is relieved by massage. Massage refreshes the muscles and one does not feel the stress of exercises or bouts.

For the very young, infants, invalids and old people, and people who are unable to do any exercise, massage is needed for proper growth and development. For growth and development their only alternative is massage.

For those who suffer from sleeplessness, self-massage or receiving massage from someone is essential each night. Foot massage is good for people who are fatigued, and for those suffering from insomnia the head should be massaged, as advised by *Charak*. Foot massage and massage of the spine is also recommended.

Massage, if executed properly, gives complete benefit of exercise. It is said by Indian wrestlers that if one only massages two persons and receives massage daily, such a person will receive the complete benefit of wrestling.

Daily practise of exercises regulates the blood circulation and increases the breath rate. The more *prana* one inhales, the more this life force from the atmosphere reaches the body. Breath purifies the blood. Increase in breath rate insures greater supply of oxygen to the deoxidised blood coming through the veins into the fine capillaries of the lungs. Breath rate which is increased by exercise strengthens the lungs. Massage, as we have described, is equivalent to exercise; in addition, it is relaxing and rejuvenating. Massage is a cleanser. The secret of youth and beauty is in the proper circulation of vital life fluids and also in the regular discharge of waste materials which, if not regularly excreted from the system, can create serious problems. Life in modern times has become very luxurious. Those who live in cities and towns do very little physical labour. Their jobs do not enable them to join in activities which would make their muscles work. This creates an imbalance in the system. Besides, they do not enjoy fresh air, natural foods or sunlight. Constant worry and unceasing anxieties create imbalance in body chemistry. The best remedy is massage. Massage as a daily practise is a must for people who are pressured with the stress and strain of modern civilisation. If daily massaging of the whole body is not possible, at least the feet should be massaged every night before sleeping; and the head could be given a massage every third day.

Massage and Exercise

Massage, if executed according to the formation of the musculature and for a sufficient amount of time, can give more benefit than exercise. The only thing to remember is that massage should be done to all the joints for a considerably longer period of time than the muscles. Rubbing-kneading-patting-striking-pressing-aqueezing of the muscles should be done simultaneously, and for as long a time as it takes for the massage area to become red and hot. This action excites the circulatory system. Massage of joints and the resultant effect under the joints accelerates the production of lymphatic fluid, purifies the blood and vitalises the organism.

Massage for Relaxation

For relaxation, massage is a fantastic device. Massage done for relaxation should be very gentle. No unbearable pressure should be applied in any way. Kneading, gentle rubbing, patting and gentle squeezing should be used. The hands should be made warm by rubbing them against each other and should be lubricated with some oil to avoid friction and uneasiness. Massage of the spine, feet and arms, shoulder muscles and the head can be enjoyed by anyone and everyone equally. Massaging pressure points relaxes the body instantaneously. If massage is done at a slow speed, and gently, it also relaxes the body very quickly. Massage done for exercise needs hard strokes and rubbing and should be done in harmony with the speed of the heart-beat; whereas massage for relaxation should be done a little more slowly than the beat of the heart.

All the day long man is engaged in unnatural activities. With ageing, one also looses the agility and quickness of youth. Physical and mental strain causes weakness in the nerves and improper circulation of vital life fluids. Tensions, constant worrying, dissatisfaction, greed and anxieties are bound to affect the organism. These enemies of mental and physical well-being bring on premature ageing. To avoid this and to help the human body and psyche, relaxation is a must. Some *yoga* postures and breathing exercises, especially deep breathing, ensure relaxation: but massage has, in addition, the miracle of touch. If this touch is soothing, massage can create wonders. Massaging daily with potent and helpful oils stops premature ageing, it provides more smartness and agility and strengthens the nerves. One becomes a person of strong nerves if one massages regularly and properly.

V
Ayurveda

In Ayurveda *(the science of Indian medicine) massage has been highly praised and people are advised to adopt it as a part of daily life.*

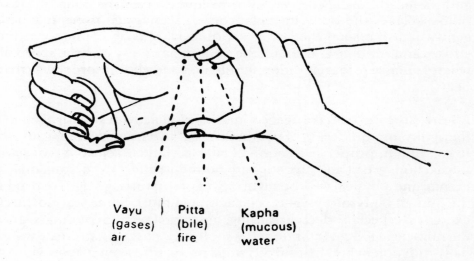

Vayu
(gases)
air

Pitta
(bile)
fire

Kapha
(mucous)
water

Marmas I

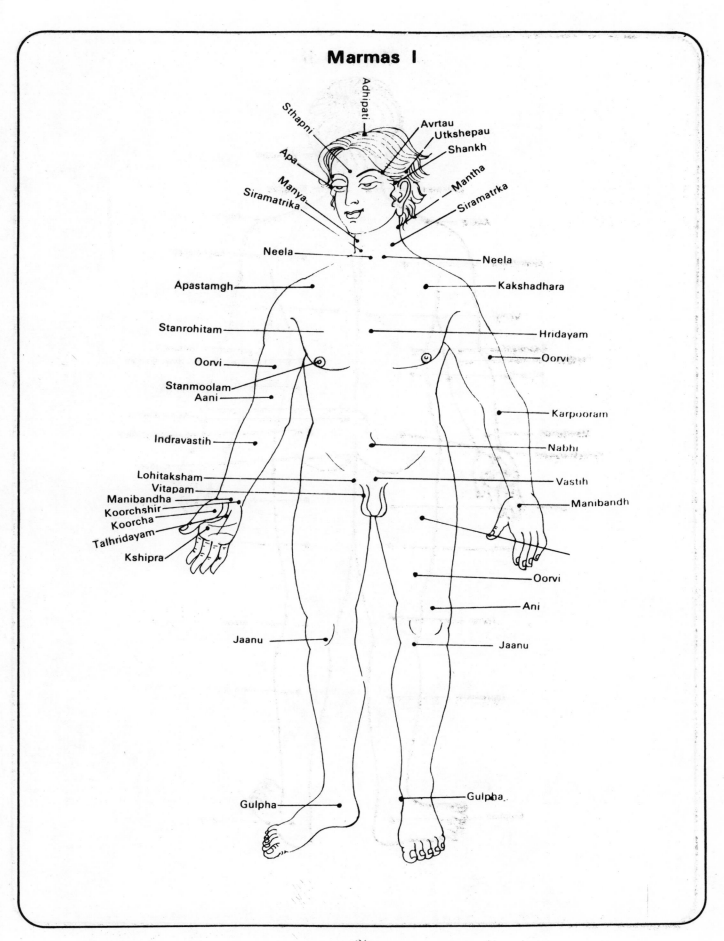

Marmas II

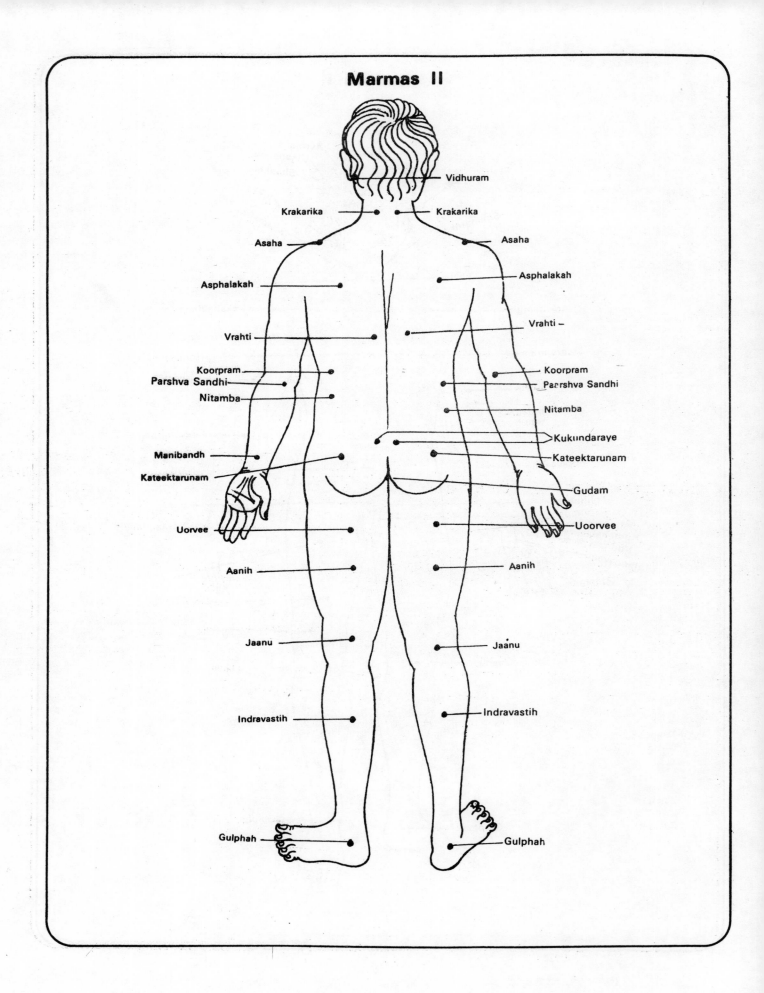

Marmas III

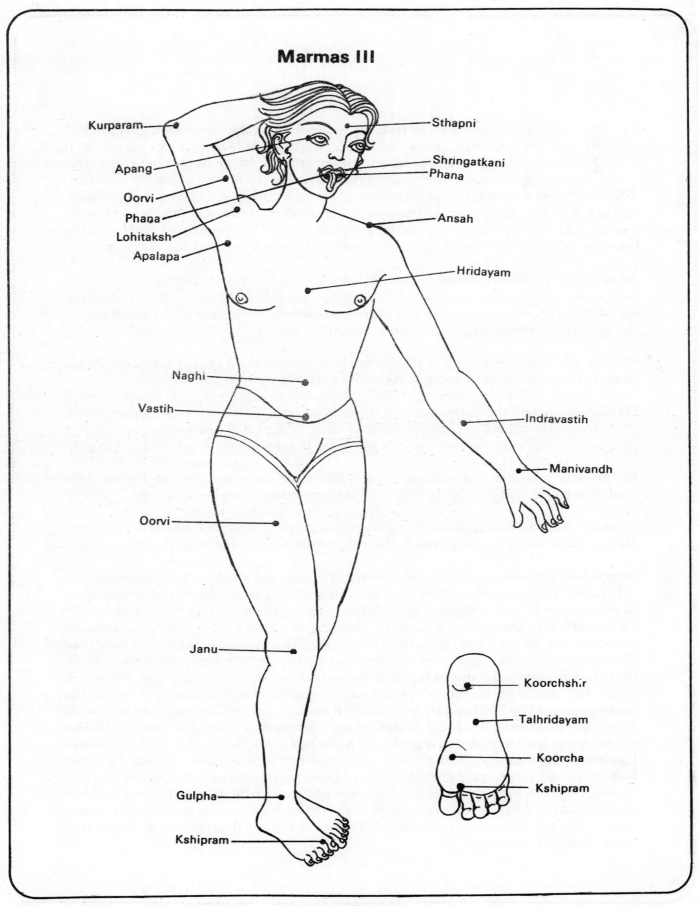

In *Ayurveda* (the science of Indian medicine), massage has been highly praised and people are advised to adopt it as a part of daily life. As we eat and sleep every day, so should we also massage and discharge our wastes every day. Massage is also used therapeutically. For different kinds of diseases, different types of massages and oil massages are prescribed. According to Vagbhatta, a writer of a famous treatise on *Ayurveda*, those who are desirous of health and happiness should massage the body, and they should use oils for massage according to the seasons. Fragrant and health-giving organic oils should be used for massage.

According to *Sushrut Samhita* (another valuable and famous scripture on Indian medicine), oil, butter or any other lubricant best suited for the body, the atmosphere and the season should be used. For persons suffering from a disorder caused by the humour of wind, massage is the only doctor.

Massage of areas specially tense should not be done without a proper lubricant. Areas having pain should be massaged for as long as one does not feel relief.

Massage increases the production of white blood corpuscles and antibodies which provide more resistance against viruses and diseases. This helps the defence mechanism in the body and increases immunity towards environmental changes.

In this way massage is a protector, preserver, and a rejuvenator, increasing self-confidence and will-power. To massage is to exercise the nervous system.

Massage plays an important role in the sexual game. *Vatsyayana,* the writer of *Kama Sutra* (treatise on sex), emphasises the role of massage in the sexual game.

In another religious scripture called *Bhavishya Purana,* the importance of massage by a wife to her husband is described in detail. It is advised that a wife should be an expert in massage. It is also recommended that massage of the waist region be done gently and slowly; the face and neck should be massaged a little harder, applying bearable pressure; but the head and feet should be massaged hardest and for a longer time than the waist, chest, face, shoulders and neck areas. Parts of the body having less flesh, thin musculature (like the navel) and important pressure points below the navel, heart, face and cheeks should be massaged gently. If the husband is awake the massage should be hard and with pressure; if he is dosing or sleeping, then he should be gently massaged like a child. Rubbing and patting only should be used and when the husband is asleep the massage should be stopped. On the parts of the body where hair grows the massage should not be done contrary to the growth of hair. To excite hair roots and to increase circulation near pores or to open up the pores, massage should be done in such a way so that the whole musculature is massaged by both hands, making cross-rhythms as shown in the figures where massage of thighs, upper legs, lower legs and arms is illustrated. The arrows in the diagram show the rhythm pattern to be followed.**

In *Ayurveda* massage is described as:

1. **Jarahar :** *Remover of old age*

   If done daily to the spine, feet and head with sesame oil, mustard oil or almond oil, massage increases virility, vitality and semen.

The body is made up of seven ingredients:

   a. **Rasa** — fluids, hormones, lymph
   b. **Rakta** — blood
   c. **Mansa** — flesh, cutis
   d. **Medha** — tendons, nerves
   e. **Asthi** — bones, teeth
   f. **Majja** — hair
   g. **Shukra** — semen

Because massage is one practice which provides energy, vitality, and nourishment to all seven *dhatus* and old age approaches late, one remains young and energetic for longer duration. In this way, massage is a remover of old age.

2. **Sharam Har :** *Remover of fatigue*

   Fatigue is actually caused by physical and mental strain. It affects the muscles and causes tensions. Rubbing, patting and squeezing muscles gently removes fatigue.

3. **Vata Har :** *Remover of the humour of wind*

   Constant strain on the nervous system from gas-producing foods and anxieties disturbs the gases and one starts having pain in the muscles and joints. Rheumatism is one of the ailments caused by wind, as is sciatica.

   Regular massage with *Mahanarayana* oil, or oils prepared by burning garlic in heated oil, or adding fenugreek seeds to boiling oil, mint oil, and wintergreen oil all help the troubles created by wind or gases.

4. **Drishti Prasad Kar :** *Increases sight*

   Daily practise of massage improves sight and keeps blindness and diseases of the eyes away. Those who have weak sight or who suffer from diseases of the eyes should massage the feet, especially under the big toe. They should also massage the spine, neck and head regularly. This will remove eye troubles and improve vision.

5. **Pushti Kar :** *Makes one strong*

   By increasing the circulation of vital life fluids, and because of rubbing, pressing, kneading, massage makes the body strong, increases stamina, vitality and virility.

6. **Ayu Kar :** *Increases longevity*
   By creating an electrochemical balance.

7. **Swapn Kar :** *Induces sleep*
   Massage relaxes the body and removes tensions. Those suffering from sleep-lessness, insomnia, or those who are unable to enjoy sound sleep should massage

the body (especially the head and feet) before sleeping. The use of oil in this case, especially oil from pumpkin seeds, massaged on the head is very helpful. *Kahu* oil is also advised. A mixture of *kahu* oil and pumpkin seed oil can be made by adding the two in equal quantities.

8. **Twak Dridh Kar :** *Strengthens the skin*
Massage makes the skin smooth and makes it shine. Regular rubbing makes it strong. Massage with oil removes dryness, which is the first sign of disturbed wind element in the body. Dryness is also caused by meditation, mental work, anxieties and constant worrying. People who live in cold climates get dry skin by constantly facing the chilled air, which creates dryness.

Wind, by nature, is cold and dry and cold is more effective when there is a cold wave or cold wind. The skin directly comes into contact with the external atmosphere, and the skin also reflects like a mirror the inner state of the physical body.

9. **Klesh Sahatwa :** *Provides resistance against disease and disharmony*
Massage excites production of antibodies and strengthens the seven ingredients of which the body is made up. These antibodies provide more resistance to disease, and the strength which comes from the seven *dhatus* gives tolerance, forebearance, and patience. This saves one from sorrows, agonies and anxieties (*klesh*)

10. **Abhighat Sahatwa :** *Resistance to injuries and power to recover quickly*
Those who massage the body regularly recover from physical injury more quickly than other persons who do not massage. The healing process from within immediately responds and comparatively less pain and fewer problems are experienced by those who massage regularly.

11. **Kapha Vata Nirodhak :** *Subsides ailments caused by mucous and wind*

12. **Mrija Varn Bal Prad :** *Provides strength to the skin and improves the colour and texture of the skin.*

Thus in *Ayurveda* massage is highly praised and much emphasis is placed on the use of oils in massage.

VI
Oil in Massage

Of All massages, those involving the use of oil are of greatest benefit.

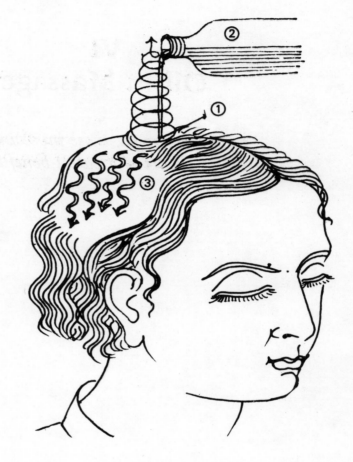

1. Twist hair-lock according to cowlick
2. Pour oil
3. Mix.

Of all massages, those involving the use of oil are of greatest benefit. Except for therapeutic reasons, the body should never be rubbed when dry, for friction, heat and pain are then produced, which in turn harm to the organism and disturb the balance of gases in the body. Patting, squeezing, kneading and striking can be done to the body if oil is not available, or if massage without oil is necessary for certain reasons. Gentle pressing or hard pressing can be done safely without oil. However, rubbing and massaging of the skin and muscles should *not* be done without oil. Oil softens the skin, lubricates it against the friction, disperses heat evenly and provides glaze, strength and resistance to extremes of temperature in the environment, as well as to sudden changes in pressure.

Oil prevents dryness, increases suppleness and durability, preventing many of the effects of premature ageing.

In India people oil their anus, genitals, nose, eyes ears, navel both as a cleansing and lubricating process—just as any machine user regularly oils his equipment to prevent the friction which can quickly ruin costly parts.

Oil is pure fire, pure caloric energy. Place a cotton wick in a cup full of oil and strike a match to the wick and the oil burns, leaving no residue. Here, in liquid form, is concentrated heat energy—fire. Oil eats friction and conducts heat readily without evaporating. Because of its quality of even distribution of heat, oil is used as a medium for cooking.

Which Oils to Use?

There are several oils which may be used in massage. Organic oils are best in all cases, for whatever one applies to the skin is in some part absorbed into the body through the pores.

Mustard Oil

Mustard oil is one of the most popular oils used for massage in north India. In the northeast, it is used as a common medium for cooking and massage. In the northwest part of India it is used for cooking, massage and it is also used by wrestlers and body-builders.

This oil is hot, unctuous, bitter, sharp and a destroyer of diseases caused by wind and mucous and it increases bile. It also increases body heat. It is a wormicide and it cures pains, swellings and wounds of all sorts. It relieves one from stiffness of muscles, from fever and bronchitis. It cleanses the blood and opens the pores. This oil extracted from yellow mustard seeds can be applied to the eyes without causing harm. No other oil is as good or as harmless as mustard oil for applying to the nose, ears, throat, anus or genitals. .It also has power to strengthen the skin and enhance pigmentation.

For patients of arthritis and gout, massage of mustard oil in which some camphor has been dissolved by slowly heating it on a low flame is recommended in *Ayurveda*.

Pain in the ears which starts suddenly can be cured by dropping a few drops of luke-warm oil into the ears.

For all sorts of swellings, massage of warm mustard oil is very beneficial. For better results, any of the following may be burned in mustard oil: garlic, asafoetida, fenugreek seeds.

Massage of mustard oil on the stomach stops enlarging of the spleen and cures it.

For any dryness, skin rash, irritation of the skin, massage with mustard oil with a small amount of turmeric powder is very relieving. Adding a little camphor or spirit of camphor is cooling and removes irritation, skin rash and itch simultaneously.

Ubtan for Beauty: *Better Shine, Colour and Glaze of the Skin*

Take fifty grams of mustard seeds (yellow or white), boil with ½ litre or 1 litre of milk and let the milk completely evaporate on a low flame, but watch that the seeds do not burn. When the milk is completely evaporated, take the seeds and dry them in the sun or any way it is possible and feasible. Make a paste out of the dried seeds and apply to the whole body. Let the paste remain on the body and relax until the paste has dried on the body. Slowly rub and remove as much of the dried paste from the body as possible. Then take a bath. Use as regularly as possible. This practise helps the skin and cures premature ageing; it increases the beauty of the skin and improves the colour and glaze of the skin. (*See also section on Beauty*)

Those who are interested in providing a natural tanning to the skin should massage with mustard oil in which some turmeric powder has been added and should then take a sun bath.

Olive Oil

Olive oil is very popular in the western world. It is used mostly for cooking and in salads, it may sometimes also be used for massage. In India olive oil is very costly because it is imported, it is only used medicinally for massage in gout, arthritis, for muscular pains, sprains and polio. *Ayurvedic* doctors and *Hakims* (those who follow the Greek system of medicine) prescribe olive oil massage. It is highly praised for being more hot than sesame oil or mustard oil. In cold climates it is very nourishing if eaten. It makes the body more receptive to solar radiation when massaged. Massage with olive oil before a sun bath could be fantastic. Olive oil is good both ways: as a medium for cooking food and making salads, and for use in massage. Olive oil is especially beneficial to children, as well as for old and weak people requiring solar energy. It is hot, unctuous, increases body heat, destroys disorders created by wind and mucous. It cures swellings and pains, relieves stiffness of muscles and enhances pigmentation.

Sesame Oil

Sesame oil is also one of the most popular oils in cooking and massage. It is most popular in the western part of India. It is used as a base for all oils used in head massage. For making oils from herbs for medical use, sesame oil is very popular amongst the *Ayurvedic* doctors. Before the discovery of white oil, sesame oil was the only oil which served as a base for all perfumed hair oils.

Sesame oil is hot, unctuous, heavy, sweet, a destroyer of disorders and diseases caused by the humour of wind, bile and mucous. Sesame oil cures swellings of all sorts and removes muscular pains and stiffness of muscles, it strengthens the skin, cures dryness of all sorts and it is very healthy for the hair. It improves the skin texture and prevents premature ageing. If massaged regularly, it improves the shape of the breasts. Massage with sesame oil increases vitality and semen. Oil of black sesame seeds is recommended in *Ayurveda* to keep the hair in good shape. It stops greying of the hair and gives back the hair its natural colour. Grey sesame seeds are medium in quality; white seeds are good for eating only. For massage, oil extracted from black sesame seeds is recommended to cure: gout, arthritis, muscle pain and swelling of any sort.

Sesame seeds contain iron, calcium and phosphorous. They also contain an enzyme which is a food for the brain and this may be one of the reasons for the use of sesame oil as a base for all hair oils. Black sesame oil absorbs more *prana* (vital life force), and is recommended for head massage and body massage. Some *vaidyas* (practitioners of *Ayurveda*) prefer sesame oil to mustard oil. Mustard oil may sometimes irritate the skin because it is pungent and bitter, while sesame oil is neutral.

Natural Oil, Mineral Oil

These oils are poor substitutes for plant-based oils, yet they are acceptable.

Baby Oil

Baby oils are generally non-organic, and invariably have synthetic aromas. They may appear to grease the hair, but really they are not providing anything to the head or the body, except temporarily removing dryness.

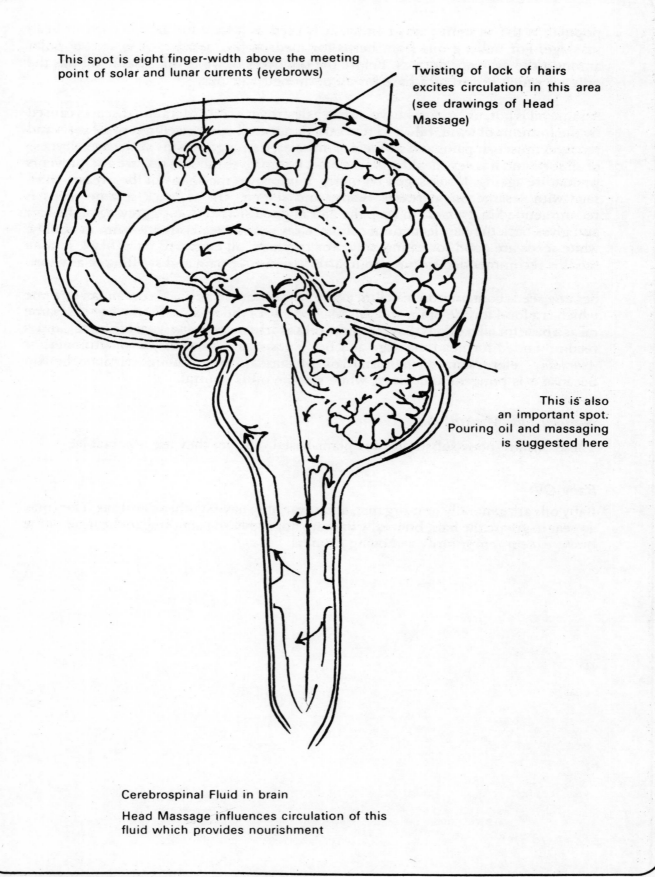

This spot is eight finger-width above the meeting point of solar and lunar currents (eyebrows)

Twisting of lock of hairs excites circulation in this area (see drawings of Head Massage)

This is also an important spot. Pouring oil and massaging is suggested here

Cerebrospinal Fluid in brain

Head Massage influences circulation of this fluid which provides nourishment

VII
Oil Formulae and Uses

For obtaining specific results different oils, herbs and spices may be cooked or mixed with the oil and different kinds of oils may be prepared. There are certain formulas which are already used by saints, folk people and Ayurvedic doctors in India. They may be used without fear.

- General
- Dryness
- Memory
- Circulation
- Young women
- Mature women
- Excess body heat
- Newly-weds and young people
- Hair—female
- Table of oils. Best Uses

OIL FORMULAS: For obtaining specific results different oils, herbs and spices may be cooked or mixed with the oil and different kinds of oils may be prepared. There are certain formulas which are already used by saints, folk people and *Ayurvedic* doctors in India. They may be used without fear.

Massage has been a favourite of kings, wrestlers, *Ayurvedic* doctors and *Hakims*. Here, we give some of the formulas obtained from them.

1. For general body massage:

To one quart of mustard oil add one ounce or ten grams of oil (not essence) of sandal wood. If there is dryness of the skin, add one ounce of wheat germ oil. For a man's massage, add a small amount of mustard oil until it smells cooked. Filter, strain and then add it to the mixture. Turmeric strengthens the skin, increase virility and heals wounds. If someone does not like the smell of mustard oil or gets irritation from it, he/she can use sesame oil using the same mixture of sandal wood, wheat germ and turmeric.

2. For dryness :

  (a) Coconut oil . . . 1 pint, plus 1 oz. wheat germ oil.

  (b) Sesame oil . . . 1 pint, plus 1 oz. wheat germ oil.

  (c) Sesame oil . . . 1 pint, plus 1 oz. almond oil and
                                     1 oz. wheat germ oil.

  (d) A mixture made from five oils:

Coconut	. . . 1 oz.
Mustard	. . . 1 oz.
Sesame	. . . 1 oz.
Wheat Germ	. . . 1 oz.
Olive	. . . 1 oz.

3. For memory:

  (a) Brahmi oil

  (b) Brahmi Amla oil

  (c) Brahmi oil   . . . 1 pint
      plus Almond oil   . . . 1 oz.

  (d) Pumpkin seed oil   . . . 1 oz.
      plus *Brahmi* or *Brahmi Amla* oil . . . 1 oz.

  (e) Mustard oil   . . . 1 pint,
      plus Almond oil   . . . 2 oz.
      plus Sandal wood oil . . . 2 oz.

4. For areas afflicted with numbness and cold and poor circulation:

  (a) Mix one dram of each: wintergreen and eucalyptus oils
              one ounce olive oil

one quart mustard oil

This mixture provides heat and stimulates the flow of energy.

(b) *Cold and chest massage:*

   (a) Heat one quart of mustard oil on a medium-high burner, adding two or more garlic cloves. When the oil is hot, allow the garlic to completely char. Let the mixture cool. Take the charred garlic out and use the mixture for massage. Warm the mixture before massage and add a pinch of salt before starting the massage. The mixture should be stored in a red bottle (cover the bottle with red paper if red bottle is not available . . . use thin tissue paper), and may be used whenever needed.

   (b) Heat one ounce of mustard oil in the same way as stated above, add 2 grams of powdered asafoetida (*heeng*), and use as mentioned above.

   (c) Heat one ounce of mustard oil and add 5 grams of fenugreek seeds in the same way as a mixture (a) above.

   (all oils used for the cure of colds of any sort should be stored in a red bottle and, if possible, should be allowed to stay in the sunlight and in an open area during the night for forty days. This increases healing power.)

5. For young women:

(a)	Black sesame seed oil	. . . 1 quart
	Jasmine oil	. . . ½ quart
(b)	Coconut oil	. . . 1 quart
	Wheat germ oil	. . . ½ oz.
	Jasmine oil	. . . 4 ozs.
(c)	Coconut oil	. . . 1 quart
	Wheat germ oil	. . . ½ oz.
	Sandal wood oil	. . . ½ oz.
(d)	Sesame oil	. . . 1 quart
	Wheat germ oil	. . . 1 oz.
	Sandal Wood oil	. . . ½ oz.
(e)	*For hair only*	
	Black Sesame oil	. . . 1 quart
	Bhringraj oil	. . . ½ quart
	Amla oil	. . . ½ oz.
	Shikakai grass powder	. . . ½ oz.

6. For women over forty years of age:

Black sesame seed oil	. . . 1 quart
Wheat germ oil	. . . ½ quart
Almond oil	. . . 1 oz.

(Massage with mixture every day.)

7. For women over fifty years of age:

Black sesame seed oil	. . . 1 quart
Coconut oil	. . . ½ quart
Wheat germ oil	. . . 1 oz.
Sandal wood oil	. . . 1 oz.

8. **For newly-weds and young couples:**

Coconut oil	. . . 1 quart
Jasmine oil (organic)	. . . 1 pint
Almond oil	. . . 1 oz.
Wheat germ oil	. . . ½ oz.

9. **For excess body heat:**

(a)
Black sesame seed oil	. . . 1 oz.
Essence of Rose	. . . 5 grams

(b)
Coconut oil	. . . 1 oz.
Pumpkin seed oil	. . . 1 oz.
Essence of Rose	. . . 5 grams

(c)
Coconut oil	. . . 1 oz.
Pumpkin seed oil	. . . 1 oz.
Essence of *Khus* (a grass)	. . . 2 grams

(d)
Sesame seed oil or Pumpkin seed oil	. . . 1 quart

Store in a blue bottle for a period of forty days in the sunlight. This oil is very cold and cures burns and bites. It also removes high fever, brings down temperature instantaneously if massaged on head and soles of feet.

(c) Use Coriander oil for massage of head and feet.

10. **For hair—female**

Bhringraj oil, *Shikakai* oil, Coconut oil . . . or a mixture of all three in equal quantities may be used.

Tables of Oils
Best Uses

Kahu oil for patients of:
insomnia and neurasthenia

Olive oil for patients of:
rheumatism, gout, arthritis and general weakness

Sandal wood oil for:
Virility and schizophrenia

Almond oil for:
brain, nervous system, weakness, old age, premature ageing and old persons

(For old people, for persons over forty-five, or for persons living in a cold climate, almond oil is very useful if taken orally in milk. One teaspoonful to one glass of warm milk taken daily anytime is a good dose.)

Babuna oil for:
muscular pains

Coriander oil for:
removal of excess body heat

Pumpkin seed oil for:
memory, insomnia, anxiety and high fever

Fish oil for:
general weakness, gout, arthritis, numbness and cold

Coconut oil for:
removing dryness, hair—female and cold feeling

Mustard oil for:
heat and vitality

Sesame seed oil for:
head and breasts

Butter, Milk, Cream of milk, (*malai*) and Beeswax for: face

Mahanarayana oil for:
rheumatism, gout, arthritis, muscular pains and polio

Seasons

Summer : Sesame seed oil

Winter : Mustard oil or Olive oil

Spring : Coconut Oil*

For sound sleep: Massage feet with oil before going to sleep at night.

For better vision : Use oil on the head in the morning.

*Women may use Coconut oil in all seasons

VIII
The Role of Vibrations in Massage

We have already mentioned the miracles of touch in massage. This should be clearly understood now: when we receive massage or when we give massage we are not only playing with the physical body, we are working with the psyche of the receiver. To understand this, we should remember one simple formula:

Energy flows from a higher level to a lower level.

The receiver surrenders himself to be massaged. He allows his body to relax and lets loose his defense mechanisms. He becomes the one who receives, who takes, and this makes him stand at a lower level. The one who receives must allow himself to absorb energy and, if one offers resistance, he will not get the complete benefit of the massage. The giver is the one who offers to give and stands on a higher level automatically. Thus as natural law, the energy is transmitted from the body of the massager to the body of the receiver. For this transference of energy the fingertips of the giver serve as a vehicle, and the skin of the receiver serves as a vehicle. There is a fine discharge of electrical energy through these fingertips and this energy is readily absorbed. Those who adopt massage as a profession and each day massage more people, they experience this loss of energy very definitely. These persons should take precautions. They should drink fresh milk or take some nuts and raisins or dates after every massage. They should also receive massage regularly and themselves relax after every massage by lying in the corpse posture for fifteen minutes. After this they should have their fingers massaged before beginning a new massage.

Wrestlers in India massage each other in order to reciprocate the process of energy transference.

After understanding the physical loss or gain of energy, one should understand that also through sympathetic response of the sympathetic nervous system there is a change in body chemistry and all fantasies and feelings are transferred to the body of the receiver.

The massager should be physically and mentally healthy. If the massager is good looking, and of soothing vibrations, massage can do miracles.

In *Ramayana,* the story of the life of *Lord Rama* (written by the first *Sanskrit* poet, *Valmiki,* in the *Ayodhya Kanda*—chapter on *Ayodhya,* the birthplace of *Lord Rama*), it is mentioned that the massage of the tired soldiers of the army of *Bharat* (younger brother of *Rama*) was done by young ladies. The description says that to refresh the soldiers, seven or eight young, beautiful girls were appointed to massage each soldier. Then they were given a bath in the river. The beautiful girls who were engaged for massage had well-built and very proportionate bodies and beautiful, pure sparkling eyes. This is sufficient to understand that the massager should be beautiful and possess soothing vibrations.

In India men generally massage men and women generally massage women—to avoid unnecessary waste of energy which can occur due to fantasising

Fantasies of sensual nature consume a great deal of energy. To avoid fantasising, the massager should concentrate on his breath, his breathing pattern and his heart-beat. A massager should raise his energy level by thinking he or she is working as a medium to transfer Divine energy into the body of the receiver. He should hold his breath while massaging. It is very helpful if young people massage old people, or if children massage old people, and if men massage men and women massage women. Children should be taught massage. They should then do it for fun. They do not fantasise, their energy is pure, and they do not suffer from loss of energy. Those who do massage as a profession should understand it, experience it, and avoid whatever does not suit them. *If massaging the opposite sex gives them no problem and sensual fantasies do not consume them, they may continue the work. If loss of energy is experienced the massager should avoid fantasizing, concentrating on the breathing pattern and keeping consciousness high.*

The massager is like a doctor and should develop immunity from body touch. He should remember while working he is playing with energy. The massager should not work when his or her energy level is down or not normal. A giver should not massage a receiver who does not vibrationally approve at first sight.

Massage is service. Service is the highest dharma. A massager should become a selfless servant and he should work egolessly.

IX
Massage and Lymph

*The Lymphatic system is the one which
is most directly involved in massage.*

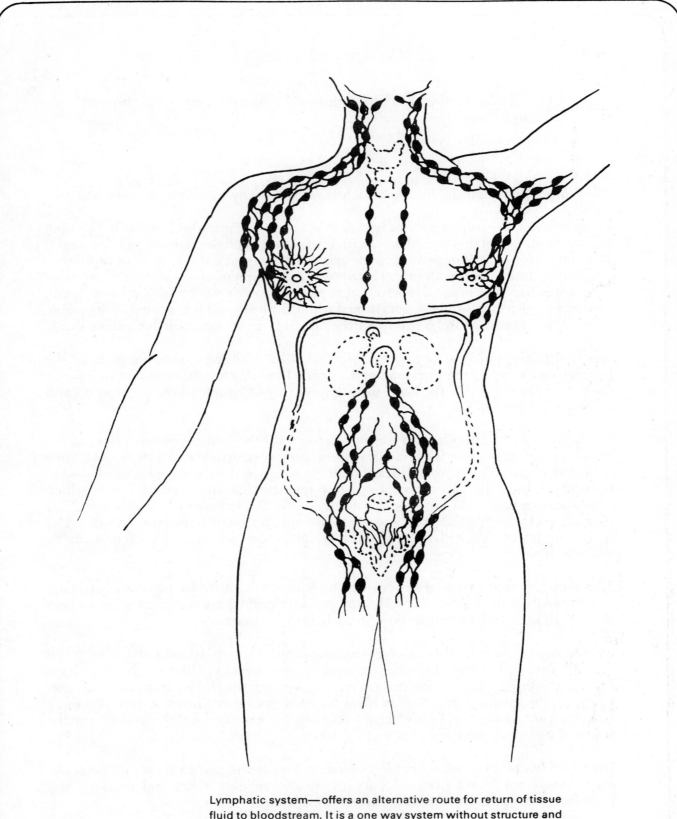

Lymphatic system—offers an alternative route for return of tissue fluid to bloodstream. It is a one way system without structure and does not form a complete circuit. They contain no valves and are unevenly distributed in body

Massage and Lymph

M assage works directly with the three circulatory systems of the human body simultaneously:

- blood vascular system
- nervous system
- lymphatic system

The lymphatic system is the one which is most directly involved in massage.

To understand the importance of lymph in massage one must look at the functioning and the functions of this complex system. It works through ducts, nodes and passages. The system is not an independent system in the sense that it does not have capillaries to carry its fluids independently. This system is a supplementary system . . . supplementary to the blood vascular system it runs side-by-side with the blood circulatory system and, through osmosis, gets mixed with the blood and is supplied to the whole body. Also, all our muscles are like fishes floating in an ocean of lymphatic fluid.

The lymphatic system assists blood circulation by draining excess liquid from the bloodstreams, easing the workload of the heart. The lymphatic system also provides a direct line of defense for the body through its army of lymphocytes, phagocytes and antibody-producing tissues.

The lymphatic system offers an alternative route for the return of tissues-fluid to the blood stream. It is a one-way system without proper structure and it does not form a complete circuit. The lymph nodes contain no valves and are unevenly distributed in the body, yet to a massager it is enough to remember that these lymph nodes (which produce lymphatic fluid) are located underneath all the joints of the body and, by rubbing and applying the circular movement, one can excite these lymph nodes. The lymph nodes are excited by local massage and heat produced by friction, or by external heat.

This complex and essential system can be stimulated more by regular exercising, compression of the individual nodes (or pressure points), by the application of heat (fomentations), and by respiration (deep breathing practises).

By stimulating lymph flow and generating heat through friction (rubbing), and through the application of the oils, massage cleanses and vitalises the body without causing the build-up of toxins and enervation which frequently accompany exercise. For this reason alone, massage is ideal for older persons whose bodies no longer readily replenish the vital fluids lost in strenuous exercise, and which can not stand the strain of age-weakened muscles and tendons.

Increased lymph flow reduces blood pressure. This is one of the reasons for prescribing massage for blood pressure patients. It also relieves aches and tensions and promotes a deeper, more natural breathing pattern.

Regular massage relaxes the system and aids digestion by maintaining a proper balance and proper circulation of gases.

X
Massage Techniques

- *Massage and the Massager*
- *How to Prepare*
- *Technique of Massage*
  - *(a) tapping*
  - *(b) kneading*
  - *(c) rubbing*
  - *(d) squeezing*

- *Post-Massage*
- *Corpse Posture*
- *Role of Vibrations in Massage*
- *Massage and Lymph*
- *Time Allotment*
- *Massage for Pregnant Women*
- *Massage for Newborn Babies*
- *Head Massage*
- *Oils to Use for Head Massage*
- *Foot Massage*

Massage is not rubbing or pressing
of the body or application of oil alone.

Massage Techniques

Massage is not rubbing or pressing of the body or application of oil alone. Many people think if they rub the body with or without oil massage is done. Ordinarily, everybody rubs his body or somebody else's body. But this rubbing and pressing is not enough. For full benefit from massage one needs to understand the systematic way of doing massage. One has to study musculature: the natural contours, the state of the three humours of wind. The massager must also study the nature of bile and mucous (whether the person being massaged has dominance of wind or gases, bile or heat, mucous or cold) in the body; when the massage should be given and when one should not massage. One must also know the role of lymph fluid in massage, the role of the circulatory system and nervous system in massage, and the role of vibrations of the massager in massage. (*It is only after understanding of the above-mentioned factors that the complete benefit can be obtained from massage*).

For the study of the natural contours and the formation of musculature one should visit any centre where human anatomy is taught and watch the formation of muscles. Or one should consult books on human anatomy and carefully study. One should study sculptures of Greek gods and develop an eye for understanding the formation of musculature. One should also study from one's, own physique.

About the three humours of wind, bile and mucous (called the three *doshas*), one should consult books on Indian medicine:

DHANWANTARI (Harish Johari, Author)
HINDU MEDICINE (Heinrich Zimmer, Author)
INDIAN MEDICINE (Julius Jolly, Author
translated into English by C.G. Kashikar)

We have made a diagram to educate people interested in ancient Indian massage from which they may learn to feel the pulse of the one receiving massage and find out which of the three *doshas* is predominant. There are also instructions pertaining to the pulse and detecting the *doshas*.

In this work also we have discussed the role of lymph fluid, which one should study and more may be studied from other available sources. We have mentioned in detail the role of the circulatory and nervous systems in massage, and in this chapter we will discuss the technique of massage and the role of vibrations in massage.

Massage in all ways increases body temperature and excites the circulation of blood in the body. This increase in the circulatory system brings toxins from all over the body through the veins to the lungs where fresh oxygen purifies the blood and recycles it in the body. This purification process and excretion of toxins can take place at the same time if massage is given in such a way that one begins to sweat. Even otherwise, these toxins are absorbed by the kidneys where the job of filtering takes place. Also, when we exhale, lots of toxins are breathed out. In the same way, massage (while working with the skin) works with the fine network of nerves lying underneath the skin and excites the nervous system. This also serves as a cleanser and provides the nerves with nourishment from within the organism.

How to Prepare:

To start massaging one needs a little preparation, the massager as well as the one receiving massage must relax before commencement. The receiver must loosen his body so that the massage does not begin in panic. For this, the receiver should first try to stand erect on his or her heels and take a few deep breaths. Then he or she should lie down on his or her back and relax for a few minutes. The giver should keenly watch the subject while he or she stands erect on the heels. He should take note of whether the receiver is indeed standing erect or whether he or she is tilting to one side. Most of the time people are tilted either to the right or to the left, believing they are standing erect. This 'witnessing' gives the massager an idea as to which side of the subject is more dominant. If the receiver is always leaning more to one side than the other, then this should be pointed out and the receiver should be asked to try to stand erect. If the receiver fails to do so, then he or she should be given more time on the opposite side and the receiver should try hard to bring himself or herself to an erect position at will. This will help the receiver in remaining mentally balanced.

Clothing should be minimal. The receiver should think about the benefits of massage while relaxing and while the massage is going on concentration should be in the particular area being massaged.

The giver, after relaxing and taking some deep breaths, should drop a few drops of oil into his palms and rub them against each other to energise the hands and to increase circulation and warmth in the hands. Then concentration should be applied as to how wonderful the healing power of massage is and wish health and relaxation to the receiver. While massaging the giver should concentrate on the areas being massaged.

The body of the receiver should be folded or turned as needed. No resistance of any kind should be applied by the receiver.

Rubbing and clapping of the hands should be repeated each time the giver removes the hands from the body or the area being massaged. This relaxes the hands of the giver, gives him time to breathe and renews his/her hands with fresh energy.

Technique of Massage

According to the traditional way of massaging, four types of strokes are used in massaging the body:

1. Tapping
2. Kneading
3. Rubbing
4. Squeezing

1. *Tapping:*

Tapping is the introductory part of massage. This awakens the body, signals are shot by the nerves. Wherever the body gets tapped, circulation increases. The body organises its defense mechanism and the person receiving the massage knows that the massage has begun. Tapping should be done with open palms and relaxed fingers. This makes the muscles strong.

2. *Kneading:*

As tapping awakens the body and increases the flow of energy into that particular area of musculature, kneading relaxes and takes out all the stress which has accumulated in the muscles during the activities of daily life. The muscles should be kneaded like dough. The massager becomes a cook, a baker, and must feel the muscles like the texture of dough in the hands. Kneading creates activity inside the cell walls of the muscles and the circulation of life-giving chemicals commences. This helps growth and development of the body and rejuvenates the body.

3. *Rubbing:*

Rubbing is the next step. There are two different ways in which rubbing is done:

- dry
- with oil

Rubbing dry, or with oil?:

Rubbing dry is an exercise for the skin, it excites circulation and increases heat in the area massaged because of friction. It also affects bones, cures stiffness of muscles and removes fatigue. *But,* it involves the danger of disturbing the gases, the wind element. Therefore, it is advised that a little oil should be used to avoid friction and to ensure equal distribution of body temperature. Rubbing underneath the joints is very useful. All lymph nodes are situated underneath the joints. Gentle rubbing helps relaxation and rubbing hard works as an exercise. Rubbing gently, making a circular movement clockwise at the pressure points, enriches the body by the release of growth hormones. Rubbing against the direction of hair growth can cause irritation. Sometimes such rubbing is therapeutic. This is a part of dry rubbing. Saints of some Hindu and Jain Orders rub ashes on their body. This creates immunity to the sense of touch and saves them from seasonal changes. The ashes become their clothes. *But, if anybody else tried to put ashes on his or her skin the skin would dry out and could cause wounds. Practices which are not commonly used and may only be made if proper knowledge of the subject is at hand, should be avoided. Anything which causes pain should be avoided.* Only gentle rubbing and rubbing with a circular movement in a clockwise direction, applying bearable pressure should be encouraged. Rhythm plays a great role in rubbing.

4. *Squeezing:*

The fourth and final step in massage is squeezing. Taking all the areas massaged once again and, with both hands, making cross movements and squeezing the whole musculature. This is done with bearable pressure and this action finally takes out all the tension and pains through the extremities—like toes in feet and fingers in the hands. While squeezing, special pressure should be applied at the pressure points. Oil should be applied in the very beginning and the giver should continue rubbing until all the oil is absorbed by the skin. Rubbing goes along with massage all the way. Squeezing is done up to the end part of the toes. When one approaches the joints of the fingers and toes one should twist the bones of the joints right and left to enhance secretion of growth hormones.

The last part in massage is the dropping of oil on the nails. After squeezing is completed, one should take a drop of oil on the fingertip and drop it on the nail in such a way so that the oil fills the gap between the flesh of the tissue on the fingers and nails.

Post-Massage

Upon completion of the massage, both the receiver and the giver should relax in the corpse posture *(The corpse posture is the rest posture which enables one to relax and to set the breathing pattern which increases with massage.)*

Corpse Posture: If one lies on one's back, putting the heals together, knees and thighs together, keeping hands close to the waist, palms open and resting on the floor, and closing the eyes one will be in the *corpse posture*. One should then concentrate on the toes, feel that they are getting numb; then think about the knees, thighs, stomach, chest, neck and head in the same manner and make them numb. After some time, when one comes again to normal consciousness, one should 'look inside' to see that there are no tensions anywhere. One should then concentrate on the *third eye* and remain in the corpse posture for a few minutes more. (*If massage is done for health and beauty, the receiver should walk very gently before lying down for relaxation.*)

Time Allotment

The decision of time duration should be taken by the giver on the spot on seeing the physical state of the receiver. If the receiver is healthy and is taking massage for relaxation and as a device to improve health, and if he or she has no pains or aches in the body the massage should not take more than thirty to thirty-five minutes. Should there be tensions, aches, pain, numbness, poor circulation, the massage should take longer. For persons who are physically weak or have a weak constitution, massage should not be long and should commence with a time allotment from fifteen to twenty minutes per session and increase to thirty or thirty-five minutes slowly.

For those who daily massage themselves, or who receive massage daily, twenty-five to thirty minutes of active massage is enough. Ordinarily, if done properly, a massage takes about forty to forty-five minutes. For infants, new-born babies, massage should be given within fifteen minutes. Old people need one hour or more for massage. From the above we see that the time factor varies from person to person.

For a clearer understanding, a chart is given below:

New-born babies	. . . 15 minutes
Infants (up to 3 years)	. . . 15-20 minutes
Young people (up to 18 years)	. . . 30-45 minutes
Healthy adults (up to age 40)	. . . 40-45 minutes
Adults (up to 60 years)	. . . According to the state of health.
Old people	. . . ,, ,, ,,
Invalids	. . . ,, ,, ,,
Patients suffering ill-health . . .	,, ,, ,,

As a principle, a giver should devote more time to areas related with sickness. For pain in muscles, massage should be given as long as the pain does not disappear.

Who should not receive Massage

One who is mucous-dominated, or one who is suffering from troubles created by aggravated *kapha* (phlegm), and one who suffers from indigestion, constipation, new fever or vomitting—such persons should *not* receive massage. Those who have taken a purgative, or who are involved with the *basti* practice of *kriya yoga* should avoid massage. Massage in such cases lowers the stomach fire and disease increases.

Massage for Pregnant Women

For pregnant women, the massage should be given very carefully, and it should be for as long a time as the woman desires. Massage can also prove to be an exertion to weak persons. In India, massage is a must for pregnant women. If properly done, it insures painless delivery. After delivery massage also is a must. Up to forty days after the fourth day of delivery, massage of the lady and the newcomer is necessary and it is done as regularly as infant and mother are given food and nourishment. Also, massage being a cleansing device, it is necessary for the mother and the child because they cannot do any exercises. There is much physical and mental strain on the body of the lady during the process of delivery. There is pain before and after delivery. Massage helps the system reorganise itself and relaxes the lady. Also, for a few months the child remains in the womb and all the musculature in the stomach region becomes mis-hapen. After delivery, message helps the body to acquire the same form as before. There are thousands of women who have four or five children and they still look like newly-married girls.

Massage for forty days after delivery is a must. It may go on as long as possible, but its duration can not be reduced. In modern times the new mothers can not afford forty days of rest. If the mother is a working woman and not a housewife, or if she is not living with other women or in a joint family, she has to work for herself, her husband and children. She can not afford forty days of rest. But, this exertion will tell upon her physical and mental health. In this modern age, where the institution of family is slowly dying, people are on one hand getting better standards of living, and on the other losing sound mental health. In this age we have to make some adjustments and we have to see how we can save our system from the sickening effects of our era. According to the Hindu system, the final purification is after forty days and before this the mother is not entitled to worship or cook and is given rest and massage every day. We can arrange at least massage, if not rest for forty days.

Massage for Newborn Babies

To massage babies is a tradition and an unavoidable phenomenon. In India, traditionally massage of the baby starts six days after birth. The massage and the cleansing of the child is done at the same time. The method adopted is very interesting: they do not massage the child with hands alone, application of oil is made with a dough ball and also rubbing the body and cleansing is all done with the help of a dough ball made of wheat flour. A dough ball—as big as a table tennis ball—is used to rub the child's body. It cleans and strengthens the child's body. The use of oil is essential and mostly mustard or sesame oil is used: in Winter, mustard oil is used and in Summer, sesame oil is used. After about thirty days really hard massage is applied to the infant, where his body becomes red and hot. The cleansing with the dough ball follows the massage and helps in r moving hair from cheeks, neck, shoulders and back.

XI
Massage for Beauty

Taking a bath with milk and rubbing of malai, cream of milk or unprocessed butter has been very popular with kings and queens in India. The skin of milk or pure cream can be tried by any girl or boy of any age group and the effect can be seen within a fortnight.

Massage for beauty starts from the base of the spine as the spine is the most important part of the body.

Massage adds glaze to the skin and increases beauty. Those who have not passed forty-five can, by using this beauty massage, become beautiful and remain looking beautiful as long as their body chemistry permits. Massage done regularly stops premature ageing and thus one remains young and energetic for a long time.

Sometimes problems, diseases and many other factors destroy the natural rhythm of the body and the body becomes dry, ugly, rough, heavy, thin, etc. At such a time certain types of massage can help. For those who are young and energetic, this massage can create miracles. This beauty massage is good for persons of all ages. If old persons (men or women) take this forty-day massage they will look younger than their age. There are certain ageing signs which appear on the face and this massage can erase those signs if one also follows the instructions as to food, etc. during and after the massage session of forty days is completed.

Massage for beauty starts from the base of the spine as the spine is the most important part of the body. If the spine is not in good shape the figure of the person will not seem right. We have already discussed the spine and here we would mention that massage of the spine can make an ugly person look graceful. The shape of one's spine is very important in looking right and one's appearance is one of the most influencing factors in beauty.

After the spine the hands are massaged, then the forearms, followed by the palms and fingers. The neck and shoulders are then massaged and lastly the head and face.

In this massage, dry rubbing is not as beneficial as application of oils, milk, cream, butter and some *ubtans* specially meant for improving skin texture.

Taking a bath with milk and rubbing *malai* (the skim from heated milk), cream of milk, or unprocessed butter has been very popular with kings and queens in India. The skim of milk or pure cream can be tried by any girl or boy of any age group and the effect can be seen within a fortnight.

One who is taking massage for beauty should use more fruits, vegetables, nuts and seeds, milk, cheese and cream during the massage period. If one starts using vegetables, nuts, seeds, etc. one week before massage commences, then one likely to get greater benefits.

Massage for beauty can not be done alone. *Ubtans* for beauty and baths can be taken alone, but for massage of neck, spine and face a giver is necessary.

The giver should make a mixture of oils for massage with the help of the following formula:

Sesame Oil	. . . 1 pint
Sandalwood Oil	. . . 15 grams
Wheat germ Oil	. . . 150 grams
Almond Oil	. . . 150 grams

Shake well, and store in the sun. This mixture should be used for massaging the spine, hands, neck and shoulders.

The face should be massaged with milk, cream of milk and special face creams of *ubtan*, the formulas for which are given below:

Soak ½ cup of lentils overnight in 1 pint of milk.
Make a paste before giving massage.

Bees-wax face cream may be used on face.

¼ glass of milk, 1 spoonful of almond oil. Mix well and massage face.

¼ cup cream, plus almond paste, plus powder of *husne yusuf* grass, powder of mustard seeds boiled and sun-dried (*see page 32*).

Other *ubtans* for beauty are mentioned under the title, *ubtan*.

The massage for beauty is a forty-day course. The massager should be a tender person and should be well-informed about the benefits of massage. All the oils and pastes involved in beauty massage should be freshly made and the massager should make them personally.

On the first day the massage should be given to the subject very gently. First, the base of the spine should be patted with oily palms, then kneading with the fingers and then rubbing should be done with wrists rubbing upwards, moving upwards with the spine. This massage should be given for fifteen minutes and then the massager and the subject should relax and talk about health, beauty, glamour, shine, glaze.

After massage of the spine comes massage of the hands. Massage of the hands should start from the shoulder blades and more attention should be devoted to the massage under the armpits, joints of wrists and fingers. The process of massage is the same: first patting with oiled fingers and application of oil, then rubbing, then kneading and moving with the musculature as shown in the illustrations on hand massage; finally squeezing the fingers and twisting the joints. Then the drops of oil should be dropped on the nails and this massage session of hands should finish. Massage should not take more than fifteen minutes—each hand. After massage of both hands, the giver and the receiver should relax.

After massage of hands comes massage of the neck and shoulders. This massage should be a little harder and should not take more than five minutes. Relaxation after this massage is not necessary.

After neck massage comes massage of the face. Formula for preparing oils or pastes have been given previously (*see page 36*). These pastes and oils or creams should then be applied to the face. The giver should at the time of applying the paste add essence of Rose. If there is facility for making cream the giver should add the essence (only a few drops) to the milk. This applies to pastes nos. 1, 3 and 4. Paste no. 4 is the best if the paste is made in paste no. 1 add paste no. 1 to paste no. 4. This paste should be rubbed on the lower jaws first and the chin and the lower jaw should be gently rubbed for about three minutes. Palms should be used and a gentle pressure should be applied. Then the massage of the cheeks should be commenced. Gentle rubbing of cheeks should be done. The giver with his or her fingers should work on each muscle. The cheeks need to be pinched, pressed and pulled. The massage of the cheeks begins from the chin and goes towards the ears and the joining part of the upper and lower jaws. All those parts where wrinkling starts with the ageing process should be lifted by the fingers and massaged. The grass *husne yusuf* is a fantastic remedy for removing wrinkles. It should be used in paste form and in cream form. It also has a fantastic aroma. Places which need attention are areas near the nose, the eyes and the lips. These places are seats of wrinkles.

Next, the nose and eyes should be gently massaged. The subject should close the eyes and the giver should gently rub the eyelids, sockets, eyeballs, and then eyebrows should be massaged; after which the massage of the forehead should start. The forehead becomes most wrinkled with age. Also, each time one thinks or faces a situation, the forehead registers the influence of thoughts and emotions. The skin should be lifted by the fingers and massaged. *Here, massage with a circular movement is very effective.*

The lips should be massaged with pure cream of milk. Cream of milk is food and can be eaten, so it will not cause any harm when it goes into the mouth. *Circular movements in a clockwise direction are very useful in massage of the cheeks, lips, nose and forehead.*

This whole work on the face should not take more than thirty minutes. Thus, this massage should be completed in about two hours, in which periods of relaxation are included.

We give below a table for clear understanding:

Spine	. . . 15 minutes
Hands	. . . 30 minutes
Shoulders and Neck	. . . 5 minutes
Face	. . . 30 minutes

So that actual massage time is 80 minutes and relaxation time is about 40 minutes:

After Spine massage	. . . 10 minutes
After Head massage	. . . 10 minutes
After Neck & Shoulders	. . . 5 minutes
After Face massage	. . . 15 minutes

The time of relaxation could be reduced, but then the results would not be the same.

Receivers of the Massage for Beauty should be advised to massage their feet or have their feet massaged before sleeping each night and also to apply *malai* or cream of milk to the face before sleeping and to wash the face with luke-warm water the following morning and to rub the face gently for ten minutes before sleeping.

Eyes are one of the most important organs in beauty. They should be washed with cold water and rose water. Rose water (not essence of Rose) is an ideal remedy for keeping the eyes clean and can provide them with more power. It is cooling and the eyes need cooling to become strong. In Nature Cure, eyes are given strength by keeping cold, wet cloths on the eyes. This also relaxes the eyes.

The finishing touch of beauty massage is given by putting a drop of rose water, having been stored in a blue bottle, into the eyes.
Kajal is very helpful to enhance the beauty of the eyes.
Kajal is made from the deposits in the *ghee* lamp (the sooty part).
Kajal is made from burning a cotton wick in cow's butter. This is the best type to use.
Kajal made from burned mustard oil is next best to cow's butter *kajal.*

While making the *kajal* from butter or mustard oil, a pinch of real organic camphor may be mixed in, this cools the eyes.
Also, a few drops of *neem* oil may be added to the mustard oil and *kajal* could be made from this mixture.

To Make Kajal:

Take some pure cotton, make a wick, dip it in the oil and burn. Put a silver plate, a saucer, a silver spoon or an ordinary metal spoon on the middle part of the flame and after a few minutes you will find carbon deposited on the plate or spoon. Scrape it onto a clean paper. Add a pinch of camphor and transfer the carbon and camphor into a small box which should be properly covered. Then pour in one or two drops of *ghee* (purified butter) and mix. If this carbon and camphor mixture is rubbed onto a bronze or silver plate with a drop or two of *ghee,* it becomes more powerful. The only point to remember is that one should rub the mixture as much as one can afford with the fingers to feel that there are no grains in the mixture. Store it in a silver box, or any box with a cover. Use *kajal* after a bath, and before sleeping—twice a day—and see how beautiful the eyes become.

There are more varieties of *kajal* and, if one is interested, one may import *kajal* from India.

The beauty massage treatment is done for forty days and the receiver is advised to continue working with cream of milk or *malai* at night and to wash the face with lukewarm water the following morning for as long as it is wise to remain beautiful. Massage of feet before sleeping should also continue. The receiver should cease wearing any kind of makeup; should cease using synthetic cosmetics.

A table for the forty-day massage and for the help of the giver; and, to obtain best possible results, the giver should follow this:

TABLE OF MASSAGE

Day	Schedule	Time	Relaxation
1st Day	Massage	80 mins.	40 mins.
2nd Day	Ubtan & Massage	80 mins.	40 mins.
3rd Day	Massage	80 mins.	40 mins.

Day	Schedule	Time	Relaxation
4th Day	Clay Bath & Massage	80 mins.	40 mins.
5th Day	Massage		40 mins.
6th Day	Massage		40 mins.
7th Day	Massage		40 mins.
8th Day	Massage	80 mins.	40 mins.
9th Day	*Ubtan*	80 mins.	40 mins.
10th Day	Massage	80 mins.	40 mins.
11th Day	Massage with Raw milk, Almond & Wheat germ oil	80 mins.	40 mins.
12th Day	Massage with Raw milk, Almond & Wheat germ oil	80 mins.	40 mins.
13th Day	Massage with Raw milk, Almond & Wheat germ oil	80 mins.	40 mins.
14th Day	Massage with Raw milk, Almond & Wheat germ oil	80 mins.	40 mins.
15th Day	Massage with Raw milk, Almond & Wheat germ oil	80 mins.	40 mins.
16th Day	Massage with Raw milk, Almond & Wheat germ oil	80 mins.	40 mins.
17th Day	Massage with Raw milk, Almond & Wheat germ oil	80 mins.	40 mins.
18th Day	Massage with Raw milk, Almond & Wheat germ oil	80 mins.	40 mins.
19th Day	Massage with Raw milk, Almond & Wheat germ oil	80 mins.	40 mins.
20th Day	Massage with Raw milk, Almond & Wheat germ oil	80 mins.	40 mins.
21st Day	Massage with Raw milk, Almond & Wheat germ oil	80 mins.	40 mins.
22nd Day	*Ubtan* and Massage	80 mins.	40 mins.
23rd Day	Massage	80 mins.	40 mins.
24th Day	Massage	80 mins.	40 mins.
25th Day	Massage	80 mins.	40 mins.
26th Day	Massage	80 mins.	40 mins.
27th Day	Massage	80 mins.	40 mins.
28th Day	Massage	80 mins.	40 mins.
29th Day	Massage of Minutes	80 mins.	40 mins.
30th Day	*Ubtan* & Massage	80 mins.	40 mins.
31st Day	Massage	80 mins.	40 mins.
32nd Day	Massage	80 mins.	40 mins.
33rd Day	Massage	80 mins.	40 mins.
34th Day	Massage	80 mins.	40 mins.
35th Day	*Ubtan* & Massage	80 mins.	40 mins.
36th Day	*Ubtan* & Massage	80 mins.	40 mins.
37th Day	*Ubtan* & Massage	80 mins.	40 mins.
38th Day	*Ubtan* & Massage	80 mins.	40 mins.
39th Day	*Ubtan* & Massage	80 mins.	40 mins.
40th Day	*Ubtan* & Massage	80 mins.	40 mins.

Ubtan for Beauty Massage:

A. Almond paste ... ½ oz.
    Cashew paste ... ½ oz
    Pistachio paste ... ¼ oz.
    Cream of Milk ... ½ oz.
    Wheat Germ Oil ... 1 tablespoonful
    Rose Water ... 1 spoonful
    Red Lentil paste ... 2 ozs.
    (Red Lentils should be soaked in milk overnight)
    Mix all the above-mentioned ingredients and check to see that the mixture has the consistency of yoghurt. Mix chickpea flour in it if the paste is too thin.

(b) Boil mustard oil seeds in 1 litre of milk and keep on a low flame until all the milk has evaporated. Dry the seeds, then powder them. (For a more detailed description see section on Oils—Mustard Oil.)
    More formulae are given in the description of *ubtan* for beauty massage.

Massage of the feet and face and the use of rose water and *kajal* should continue.

A bath with rose water should be taken after each session, with *ubtan* and raw milk massage.

A sun bath for people who live in cold climates during this treatment is marvellous. The sun bath should be taken after massage, during the period of relaxation.

The hair should be washed with soap-nut powder, *amla* powder, chickpea flour, clay, yoghurt, buttermilk or raw milk—as suits the subject.

During the 21-day raw milk massage session, commencing with the 11th day and ending with the thirty-first day, three or four times (or more if possible) the hair should be washed with raw milk. Fresh milk from the cow should be obtained for this, and the receiver should be advised to fast once or twice a week—drinking only milk and fruit juices during the fast.

The use of tobacco, alcohol, meat, fish, eggs or any non-vegetarian food should be avoided.

XII
The Cleansing Massage

Ubtan

Application of ubtan cures disorders caused by imbalance of mucous. It increases semen, enhances strength and stamina, stimulates circulation and cures diseases and infections of the skin. The use of ubtan on the face relaxes the jaws and neck muscles and provides a healthy, clear complexion.

Indian folk healers have evolved a practise which combines the best elements of cleansing the body with all the benefits of massage. This is known as *ubtan*.

Ubtan is commonly used in north India and is made in so many ways. We have already mentioned a few, while writing about Beauty Massage. Some more formulae are given below:

For General Body Massage:

Mustard oil	. . . ¼ oz
Chickpea flour	. . . 2 ozs.
Turmeric powder	. . . 1 teaspoonful

Make a thick paste, add water (as much as is necessary).

For Skin Growth, Smoothness and Glaze:

Mustard oil	. . . ¼ oz.
Chickpea flour	. . . 2 oz.
Turmeric powder	. . . 1 teaspoonful
Fenugreek powder	. . . 1 tablespoonful

Add water to make a paste.

For People Suffering from Rheumatism:

Olive oil	. . . ¼ oz.
Fenugreek powder	. . . ¼ oz.
Mustard oil	. . . ⅛ oz.
Garlic powder	. . . ¼ teaspoonful
Chickpea flour	. . . 2 oz.
Turmeric powder	. . . 1 teaspoonful

Add water to make a paste.

For Pimples:

Chiraunji paste	. . . ¼ oz.
Dried skin of orange powder	. . . ¼ oz.
Coconut oil	. . . ¼ oz.
Wheat germ oil	. . . 1 spoonful
Turmeric powder	. . . ½ spoonful
Chickpea flour	. . . 1 oz.
Organic camphor (powdered)	. . . pinch

Ubtan is a paste and should be applied to the skin. The one applying *ubtan* should relax till the paste begins drying on the body. The moment it starts drying, rubbing of that area and taking off the paste should be started. The removed paste can be made into a ball. Rubbing with that ball helps remove the remaining paste from the body as well as dirt from the body. This rubbing with the ball opens all the body pores and provides nourishment to the body. The fine parts of the chemicals and oil are also absorbed by the skin which then go inside the body and strengthen the nerves. Friction and rubbing to remove the paste increases circulation of blood and provides energy.

Application of *ubtan* cures disorders caused by imbalance of mucous, it increases semen, enhances strength and stamina, stimulates circulation and cures diseases and infections of the skin. The use of *ubtan* on face relaxes the jaws and cheek muscles, and provides a healthy, clear complexion.

As soap is the greatest enemy of the skin by its action of stripping the much-needed natural oils and chemicals away and dessicating the pores, so is *ubtan* the greatest friend and cleanser. The turmeric added to the mixture provides iodine in a form which can be absorbed by the skin, stmulating the nerves throughout the system. The oil and flour both cleanse and lubricate and they create smoothness and glaze as well as a healthy glow to the skin.

The initial application of the paste draws heat out of the system. The rubbing, which begins afterwards, restores normal temperature and draws fresh energy to the surface of the entire organism. Then rubbing with the dough ball increases body heat and blood circulation. Thus, *ubtan* is a cure-all for the disorders caused by the humour of wind, bile or mucous. It establishes a balance in body chemistry.

XIII
Therapeutic Massage

- Sprains or Dislocation of Bones
- General Weakness
- Rheumatism
- High Blood Pressure
- Paralysis
- Insomnia
- Arthritis
- Neurasthenia
- Sciatica
- Polio

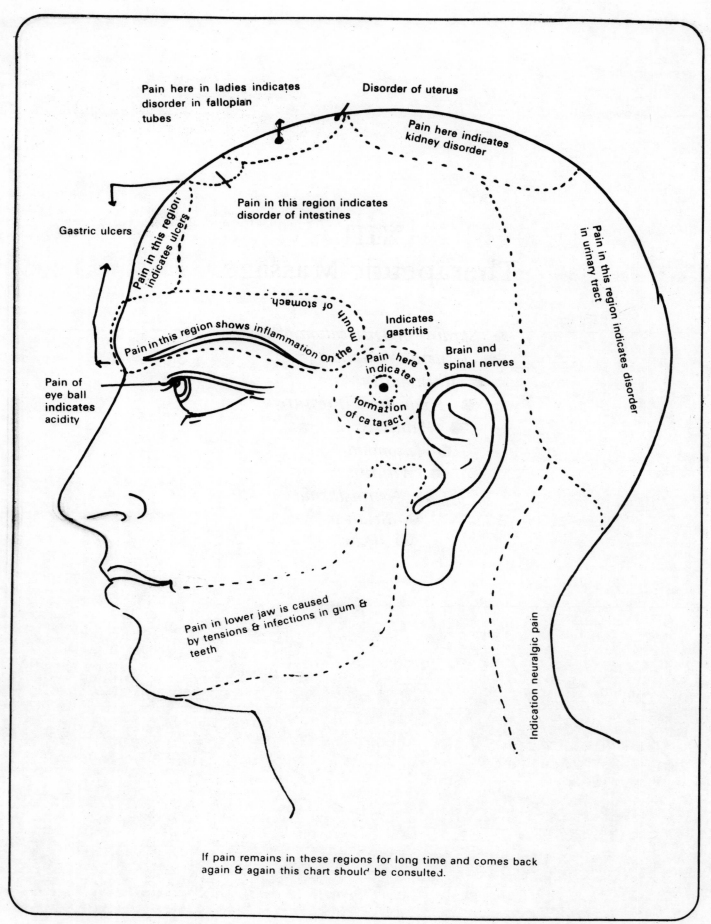

Pain here in ladies indicates disorder in fallopian tubes

Disorder of uterus

Pain here indicates kidney disorder

Gastric ulcers

Pain in this region indicates disorder of intestines

Pain in this region indicates ulcers

Pain in this region indicates disorder in urinary tract

mouth of stomach

Pain in this region shows inflammation on the

Indicates gastritis

Brain and spinal nerves

Pain here indicates formation of cataract

Pain of eye ball indicates acidity

Pain in lower jaw is caused by tensions & infections in gum & teeth

Indication neuralgic pain

If pain remains in these regions for long time and comes back again & again this chart should be consulted.

62

1. *For General Weakness:*

In childhood, after a long ailment, and in old age, this massage is needed. Massage as described in the technique of massage. Use:

    (a) Olive oil
    (b) Almond oil, or
    (c) Fish oil

Make a mixture with oil from black sesame seeds with any one of the above-mentioned three oils if these oils in pure form are in any way not suitable.

2. *For Sprains or Dislocation of Bones:*

    (a) Mustard oil   . . . 1 oz.
         Iodex   . . . 1 teaspoonful
         Mix, and massage the affected area.
    (b) Mustard oil   . . . 1 oz.
         Powdered turmeric   . . . 1 spoonful
         Mint oil   . . . 10 drops
         Iodex   . . . ½ teaspoonful
         Fomentation with water bottle, or warm oil helps.
         Application of a cloth strip, coated with clay paste, helps.

3. *Arthritis:*

Pain in arthritis is caused by poor circulation in the joints. For a better degree of circulation in that area the affected part should be given fomentation with warm water for about three minutes. The one-minute application of cold water should be done, then the fomentation with hot water should be repeated. After this, massage with a mixture of olive oil (1 oz), mustard oil (1 oz), wintergreen oil (10 drops), eucalyptus oil (10 drops), and mint oil (10 drops). Shake well and warm the mixture before giving the massage. This will increase circulation. After massage, tie a cloth strip coated with clay paste on the afflicted area. Let it remain for approximately forty minutes. This treatment applied for forty days will help.

4. *Rheumatism:*

In this disease the maximum pain is experienced in the joints. Joints are the areas where blood vessels have to take a turn, and it is natural that waste material gets clogged near the joints. Also, with the increase of acidity in the blood, one suffers from diseases caused by the impurities of blood. The digestion becomes poor and one suffers from indigestion, constipation, gases, etc. To balance the body chemistry cleansing massage, sweating, enema and hard massage are needed. The toxins deposited near the joints cause rheumatic pain. And, as long as these deposits remain, health can not be brought back. Steam fomentations on the back, sweating, massage—the three combined—can do miracles.

    Use (a) Olive oil for massage
         (b) Mustard oil for massage

(c)   Fenugreek powder paste on affected area.
      (Put paste on a strip of cloth and tie it on.)
(d)   Mustard oil in which garlic cloves have been charred.
(e)   Fish oil, with mustard or sesame oil.
(f)   Oil from red bottle.
(g)   *Babuna* oil.
(h)   *Mahanarayana* oil.
(i)   Mixture of *Mahanarayana* oil and *Babuna* oil.

5. *Neurasthenia:*

This disease is mental and the cause is weakness of mind (brain and nervous system). The patients complain of back-ache, pain at the waist region especially. Sometimes they experience a burning sensation. Their blood capillaries become weak and this influences their mind. They lose the power to make decisions. They become very fickle and lose self-confidence, faith in themselves and in others. They always think negatively about themselves and others and sometimes they suffer from persecution mania. Constant worrying, anxieties and restlessness also causes this disease. These factors, i.e. anxiety and restlessness, increase the disease more and more. Such persons are easily excited. They are afraid and extremely jealous. Excess of this can cause them to distrust the world and increase suicidal tendencies. The patients of neurasthenia become nervous very quickly and sometimes they become psychotic, neurotic, crazy and ultimately mad. They live under constant tension and need more attention. Excess indulgence in sexual games and wasting energy by fantasising also causes this disease.

For such patients, massage is a must. They need to improve circulation of blood, their digestion and they need relaxation and good diet; also more milk, yoghurt, salads, fruits, vegetables and rest. Rubbing hard, pinching, squeezing, patting, etc. helps while massaging. Use of oil is very helpful. Exercises in the morning. Bathe with luke-warm water in winter and water at room temperature in summer after one hour of massage. Cold water strengthens nerves. Massage of the back with warm and cold oil simultaneously helps. The back should be heated with a hot water bottle, then massaged with a cold towel. Sun bath and morning walk help.

Use *kahu* oil, almond oil and sandalwood oil . . . 1 oz. each. Add to one quart of mustard oil and one tablespoonful of turmeric powder. Massage daily. Take a sunbath first, then bathe. Getting up before dawn and taking a walk in the morning help.

6. *High Blood Pressure:*

Massage in the case of blood pressure is a very effective remedy, but it should not begin from the head and move towards the feet. Gentle massage with light pressure is prescribed. Massage with cooling oils is very helpful. Luxurious living, fatness, laziness, lack of physical exercise, fried foods, excess of fat, oils and ghee in the food, smoking, or drinking liquor—whatever may be the cause of this disease, the cure is one: purification of the blood vessels, by drinking more liquids, especially water, massage and a balanced diet.

Constriction of the blood capillaries makes the heart use more power to send blood to the entire body and this causes the high blood pressure. The patient must control his habits: leave intoxicants and tobacco out of his diet. He must do physical labour. It is necessary to consume more fruits, fruit juices and vegetables (raw or boiled, as necessary). The use of sesame oil or mustard oil is good—whichever suits. Jasmine oil or Rose oil can be used if the patient likes either one. In the case of blood pressure, the whole body should be regularly massaged with oil.

7. *Sciatica:*

This nerve is located at the waist region, from there it goes through the thighs and to the ankles and then to the feet. Because of certain reasons this nerve becomes tense. Pain sometimes appears. In the illustrations on foot massage we have specially marked the areas in the ankles and feet relating to this nerve. Massaging the areas marked helps cure sciatica. Heat is needed. More rubbing at the point of pain near the hip bones, waist, thighs and ankles is needed. A sun bath, or massage in sunlight helps. Use a strip of cloth coated with paste made from fenugreek powder and applied to the afflicted area also helps. Use a hot water bottle; oil from a red bottle; red rays of light. Rubbing, kneading, and rhythmic massage help. Use of fenugreek seeds and garlic in food also aid. *Arnica* oil, *Mahanarayana* oil and oil made by charring fenugreek seeds in mustard oil help.

8. *Paralysis:*

Whatever may be the cause of paralysis, massage of the afflicted area helps. The areas affected by paralysis suffer from poor circulation of blood. Massage, as we know, enhances circulation, the only thing to remember is that a patient of paralysis needs massage for a very long time. And, as such, massage should be done many times during the day. Almond oil, olive oil, mustard oil, fish oil, oil made from fat of pigeon and hot and cold massage done simultaneously help the Massage with *Mahanarayana* oil helps, as do sun baths and good diet.

9. *Polio:*

Polio is basically a disease of children. In addition to other causes, one cause is poor circulation. Massage helps to cure polio. Massage should be done at least four times per day—in sunlight. After massage in the sunlight the patient should go in a hot tub for three minutes and then for twenty minutes the patient should be given hot and cold fomentations simultaneously. Fish oil should be used for massage. Patience on the part of the receiver and the giver is required. Months of massage may show some improvement. Use of garlic in food and massage with *Mahanarayana* oil both help.

10. *Insomnia:*

Sleeplessness, disturbed sleep, is a boon of the industrial civilisation. Massage of the feet before sleeping and massage of the head with pumpkin seed oil or *kahu* oil, or a mixture of the two in equal quantities helps. This disease, if it is allowed to continue for a longer time, can cause a nervous breakdown. The rhythm pattern of the body gets disturbed by acting contrary to the laws of nature. Not getting up before dawn, waking up at night, being employed in an uninteresting job, irregular habits, anxieties, constant stress and strain are the main causes of this disease.

People who do not do any physical work and work only with the mind suffer from this ailment. Mental fatigue causes disturbance in the nervous system and such persons can not relax or sleep. Tobacco smoking, eating late at night, reading exciting literature, living in a closed apartment, palpitation of the heart, guilt feelings, and excitement also cause insomnia.

Music of *Tamboura* (Indian musical instrument) *tuned for the time of day is a cure.*

CHARAK gives a vivid description of sleep:

> "All pleasures and pains, health and disease,
> vitality and weakness, growth and decay, wisdom
> and ignorance—even life and death—come to us
> through sleep."

You sleep all right, when you wake up you feel sickness has crept inside you while you were asleep. Our sleep can be categorised as:

Sleep produced by *tamas.*
Sleep produced by increase of mucous in the body.
Sleep produced by physical or mental strain.
Untimely sleep.
Sleep produced by disease.
Natural sleep.

Natural sleep comes at night. Because of the position of the planet, Earth, the effect of gravity, this sleep is divine: it cleans the garbage from the mind, improves health, stamina, vitality, wisdom and it improves our knowledge. In this natural sleep the body reorganises itself through dreams. People have visions in dreams. Only this sleep is genuine. Other types of sleep, as we have seen, are because of increase in *tamas;* they are unnatural.

In *Sushruta-samhita* (treatise on *Ayurveda*) sleep is described and it is said that patients of humour wind are the ones who suffer mostly from insomnia. Lack of physical work and exercise causes disturbed sleep. Patients of insomnia should do some physical labour. They should avoid sleeping at unnatural times. One should never sleep during the day, except in hot countries and in summer. Morning walks help cure this disease. Massage of the back and head especially helps. Massage for insomnia should always be done by someone liked or revered by the patient. Self-massage does not help much. Sun baths help. Hot and cold baths, given simultaneously , help.

One thing should be remembered: the head should *not* get any heat. The head should be washed in normal room-temperature water and then a wet towel should be wrapped around the head before the patient takes a hot water bath for two minutes, then a cold-water bath of two minutes' duration. After the bath fifteen minutes of relaxation is necessary. This bath should be given to the patient *after* massage.

XIV
Practical Guidance for Massage

We have already discussed the sequence of massage in the chapter of the Sequence of Massage, for our readers we are providing here diagrams and practical guidelines for massage. Those who are interested in working with massage should carefully study the chapter which deals with how to prepare for massage and then follow the method which is given here in the illustrations.

Massage can start from the base of the spine or feet. In India both systems are popular. Those who start the massage with the feet gradually move from—the feet . . . to the calves . . . knees—thighs . . . upper legs . . . hips . . . and then work on the back—and front of the torso . . . after back they massage the hands (the arms)—and in the end they massage the head. Those who start from the base of the spine . . . work on the hips . . . simultaneously—and then go down to the upper leg . . . thighs . . . knees . . . calves . . . ankles—and finally finish with the foot massage. Then they come back to the base of the spine—and start the massage of the back and front of the torso—and then work with the arms and hands. In the end they do the head massage—and finish the massage. We have found the system which starts with the base of the spine and proceeds down to the feet more effective—and shall provide practical guidelines for this way of massaging only.

Massage is working with hands—and with breath, the massager should work with the rhythm of one's own heart beats. One should not do any strenuous work on the body. The pressure applied by the massager should be bearable otherwise the body will have to produce resistance in order to bear the pressure. However massage should not be too gentle otherwise the people getting massage will start fantasising—and get into a semi-hypnotic state.

The massager should relax his hands—by shaking them gently moving the wrist and palms in a circular movement . . . or by making mudras rhythmically . . . In the end one should move the hands faster . . . and shake them in a relaxed manner until one feels a tingling sensation in the fingertips . . . Now the fingertips are charged with fresh energy—and are ready to start the first step of tapping. The person going to be massaged should be asked to lie down on his stomach . . . keeping the arms the way one feels comfortable.

Start the massage with Tapping. Tapping is giving a signal to the body that massage is starting. Keep your palms open, and fingers relaxed.

After Tapping start kneading gently the lips—and press them gently . . . kneading and pressing goes together. Pressing also excites the fine capillaries of the blood vescular system—as tapping does, but in pressing one stops the flow of blood through them. After the pressure is removed the blood which has been stopped rushes forward with greater pressure—and the circulatory system gets cleaned.

After kneading shake the muscles, using both the hands on either side of the muscles —spread oil after the muscles are relaxed.

Hip and Side Massage

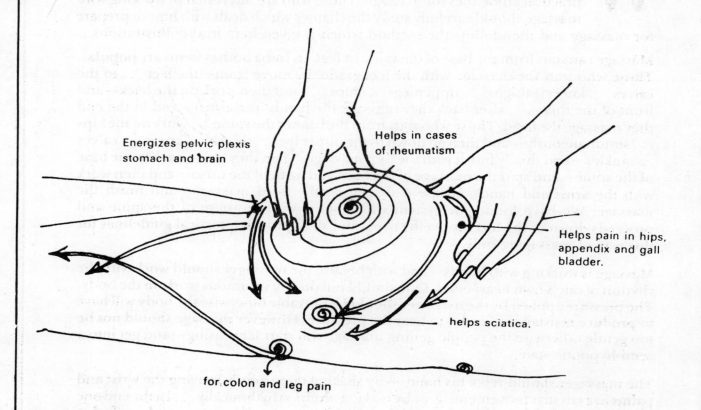

Energizes pelvic plexis stomach and brain

Helps in cases of rheumatism

Helps pain in hips, appendix and gall bladder.

helps sciatica.

for colon and leg pain

Hip and Side Massage

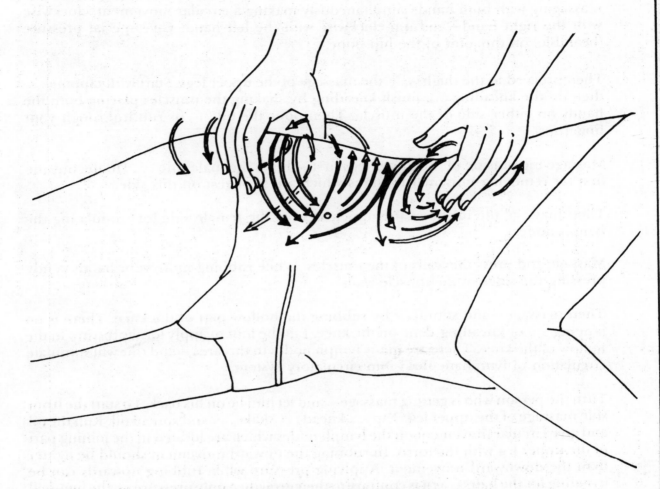

This massage helps stomach, intestines, waist region, pelvic plexis, hypo gastric plexis, colon, liver, spleen and all tensions. It is very relaxing and energizing.

Massage of the Upper Leg

Fix your thumbs on the base of the spine (ending part of the pelvic region). With fingers rub the pressure point at the joint of the hip bone. Start rubbing the oil and massaging with both hands simultaneously making a circular movement, clockwise with the right hand—and anti-clockwise with the left hand. Give special pressure (bearable) on the joint of the hip bone.

Then proceed to the thighs . . . the massage of the upper legs. Start with tapping . . . then do the kneading . . . finish kneading by shaking the muscles placing both the hands on either side of the muscle. Then pour the oil . . . or rub it through your fingertips.

Massage the outside of the upper legs first—this is the male side . . . Do the outside first for removing muscular tensions which are strongest on this side.

Then massage the inside of the upper legs . . . the female side for stimulating the lymph nodes.

Massage and press the walls of the muscles. While rubbing more your hands gently pressing the sides of the muscle walls.

Then massage—and stimulate by rubbing the hollow part of the knee. There is no tapping . . . or kneading done on the knee. Lift the foot to apply local pressure in the hollow of the knee. There are many lymph nodes in this area—and this will stimulate circulation of lymphatic fluid into circulatory system.

Turn the person who is getting massage—and let him lie on his back. To start the front side massage of the upper leg. Tap . . . knead . . . shake . . . and spread oil. Rub the oil and give circular movement on the lymph nodes which are located in the joining part of the upper leg with the torso. In rubbing the upward movement should be lighter than the downward movement. Applying pressure while rubbing upwards can be irritating for the hairs—as it is contrary to their growth. Apply pressure on the inguinal lymph nodes. Lift the knee to reach the other side of the upper leg.

Then massage downwards from knee to the ankle.

Upper Leg Massage

(outside of leg)

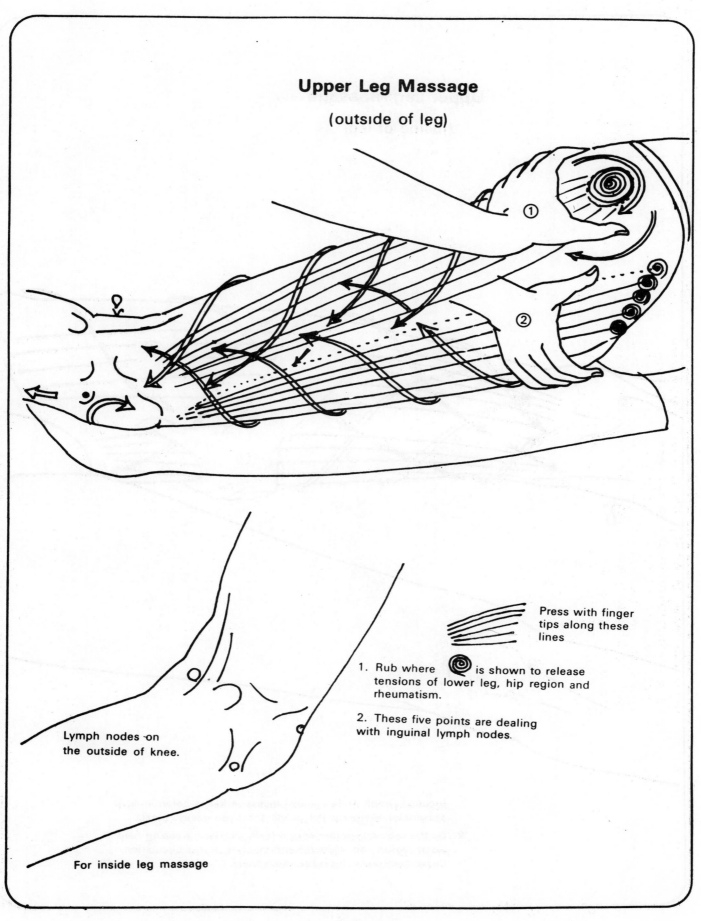

Press with finger tips along these lines

1. Rub where 🌀 is shown to release tensions of lower leg, hip region and rheumatism.

2. These five points are dealing with inguinal lymph nodes.

Lymph nodes on the outside of knee.

For inside leg massage

Upper Leg Massage

(Inside of leg)

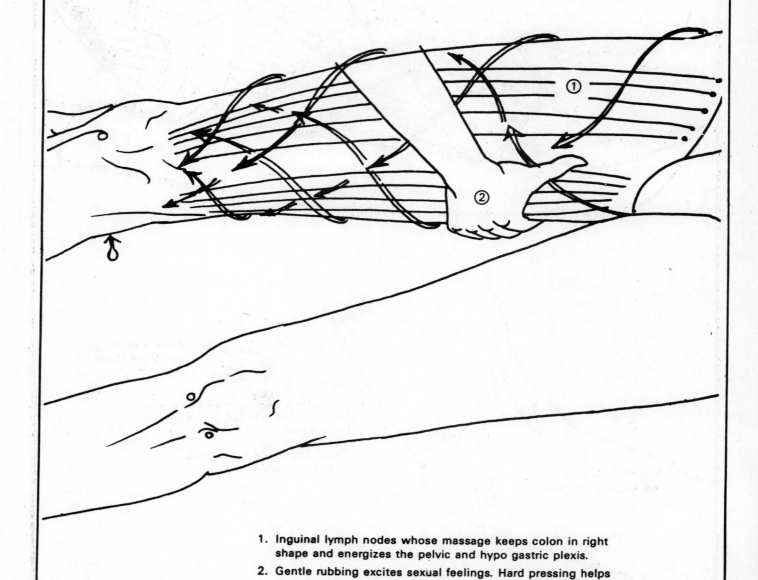

1. Inguinal lymph nodes whose massage keeps colon in right shape and energizes the pelvic and hypo gastric plexis.

2. Gentle rubbing excites sexual feelings. Hard pressing helps waist region and adductor and magnus. Helps circulation. Cures numbness. Increases sensitivity.

Massage of the Lower Leg

There are four points on the knee where the pressure should be applied. To apply pressure—and work with this area one should hold two points by thumbs of both the hands—and the two fingers (forefingers) should be placed in the hollow area of the knee near the tendens. The thumbs should be placed in a way that they are holding the two alternate points—and are not to be placed parallel to each other. One thumb should be placed on the lower part of the knee cap—and the other on the other side on the higher side of the knee cap . . . The fingers which are on the other side of the knee cap, in the hollow area near the tendens should remain tightly pressing the pressure point near tendons—and with the thumbs one should make circular movement . . . clockwise with the right hand—and anticlockwise with the left hand. One should then change the position of the thumbs, by reversing the order, and covering the other side of the knee-cap.

After this the hollow area of the knee should be rubbed in a little faster rhythm—and the massage of the lower leg should be started.

For massaging the lower leg the foot should be raised and placed on the knee of the massager. The foot should be placed in such a way that the muscles of the calves are completely loose. Tapping, kneading and shaking should be done in proper order —and then oil should be applied. There are three important points here in this area of calves—as shown in the diagrams. The two points on the sides should be given pressure and should be rubbed making a circular movement as shown in the drawings. After this the massager should work with the calves. He should make the shape of his palms like a cup—and start rubbing the calves alternately with both hands in a fast rhythm.

The massage of the lower leg finishes with the rubbing of either side of the area of the ankle joint, just above the heels. This area is of vital importance and the famous nerve Ischias passes through this area.

Start the massage of the foot by relaxing the foot through a circular movement—clockwise for the right foot and anticlockwise for the left foot.

Lower Leg Massage

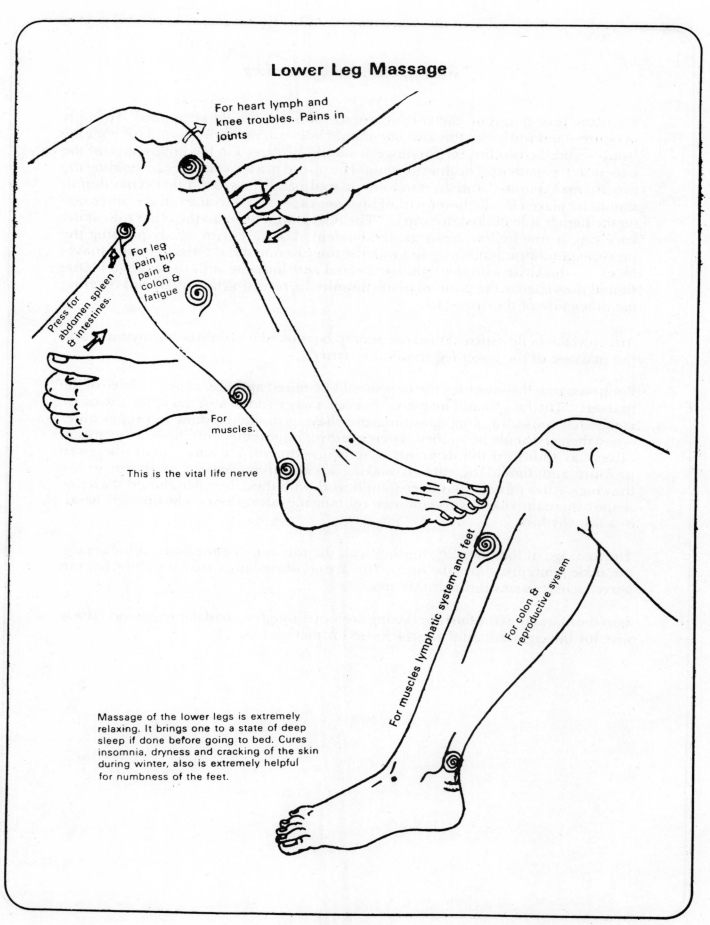

For heart lymph and knee troubles. Pains in joints

For leg pain hip pain & colon & fatigue

Press for abdomen spleen & intestines.

For muscles.

This is the vital life nerve

For muscles lymphatic system and feet

For colon & reproductive system

Massage of the lower legs is extremely relaxing. It brings one to a state of deep sleep if done before going to bed. Cures insomnia, dryness and cracking of the skin during winter, also is extremely helpful for numbness of the feet.

Foot Massage

Foot massage is highly praised in *Ayurveda*. There is nothing more healing and effective than a foot massage before sleeping. *Vishnu* is always shown reclining in his serpent coil getting a foot massage from his wife, *Lakshmi*. This *Vishnu* is the Lord of Preservation. Foot massage really preserves man from disease and troubles and brings peace, prosperity and good luck. According to Indian scriptures: *"Diseases do not go near one who massages his feet before sleeping, just as snakes do not approach eagles."*

It is said that the soles of the feet contain end parts of all the organism, and there are connections with the soles of the feet and the various organs of the body. In classical drawings of the feet, all these energies are represented by symbols. Feet discharge energy and worship of the Lotus feet of the teacher or *guru* is highly praised in *Tantra* and *Yoga*. In *Shaktipat Maha Yoga* (*Yoga* of transference of energy) the *guru* opens the path of *Kundalini* by transferring his energy into his disciple by hitting him through his Lotus-feet.

A simple mustard oil massage of the feet prevents cold weather cracking and peeling of skin, it reduces and eliminates infections caused by fungus and bacteria and reduces agitation and also promotes sound sleep.

Pouring oil in drops on the nails stops hardening of the nails, cracking of the nails and makes the nails shiny and beautiful.

Work on all the joints . . . press . . . them because no tapping, kneading or shaking is to be done in this area.

Then hold the foot from the backside—placing the thumb on one side of the joint which is in the area of the ankle bone and the forefinger on the other side of the foot at the juncture of the foot with ankle bone on the rear side. Then with the other hand start massaging the foot. The thumb should always be placed on the joining point on the front side of the ankle bone and the fore finger on the joining point on the rear side. If these points are rightly pressed simultaneously it will numb the foot on the side of the thumb. This shows that circulation gets blocked on one side through this method . . . and the massage is performed by the other hand on the side which does not get numb. After this blocking one side —and massaging the active side the massager should alternate the positions of the thumbs—and the forefinger, blocking the circulation on the other side . . . and massaging the side which was blocked before. The massager should always as a principle first massage the outside and then the inside.

Then rub the heels in a fast rhythm to increase circulation. After this start massaging the sole of the feet. See the diagram, soles of the feet are of vital importance because of their relationship with internal organs of the body.

Massage the soles thoroughly. Each joint should be properly articulated.

Turn the foot . . . press it from the front . . . then hold it again with one hand and move

Foot Massage

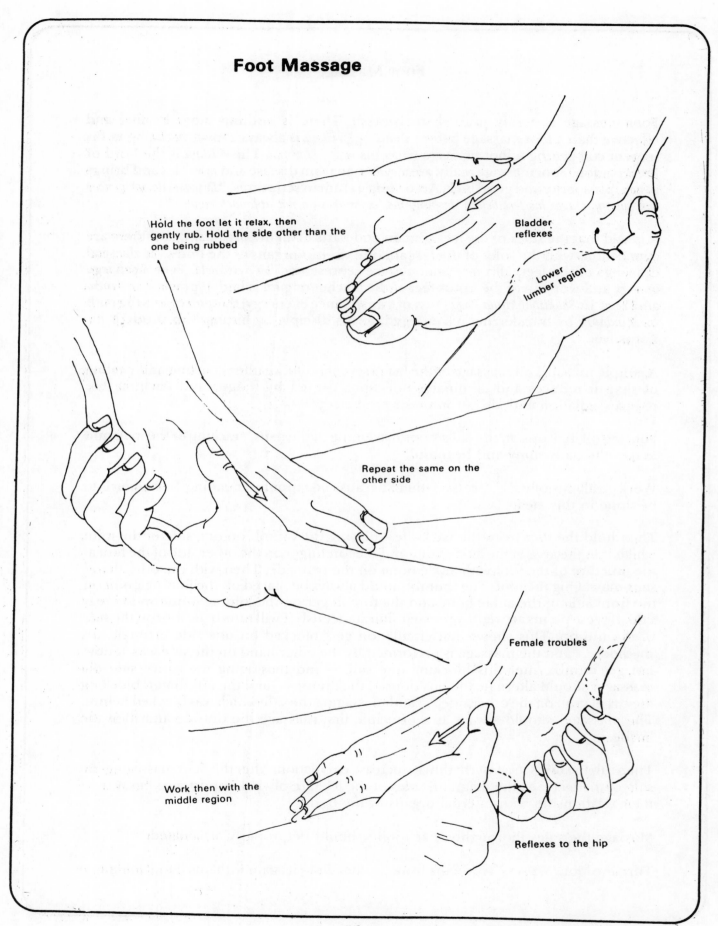

Hold the foot let it relax, then gently rub. Hold the side other than the one being rubbed

Bladder reflexes

Lower lumber region

Repeat the same on the other side

Female troubles

Work then with the middle region

Reflexes to the hip

Foot Massage

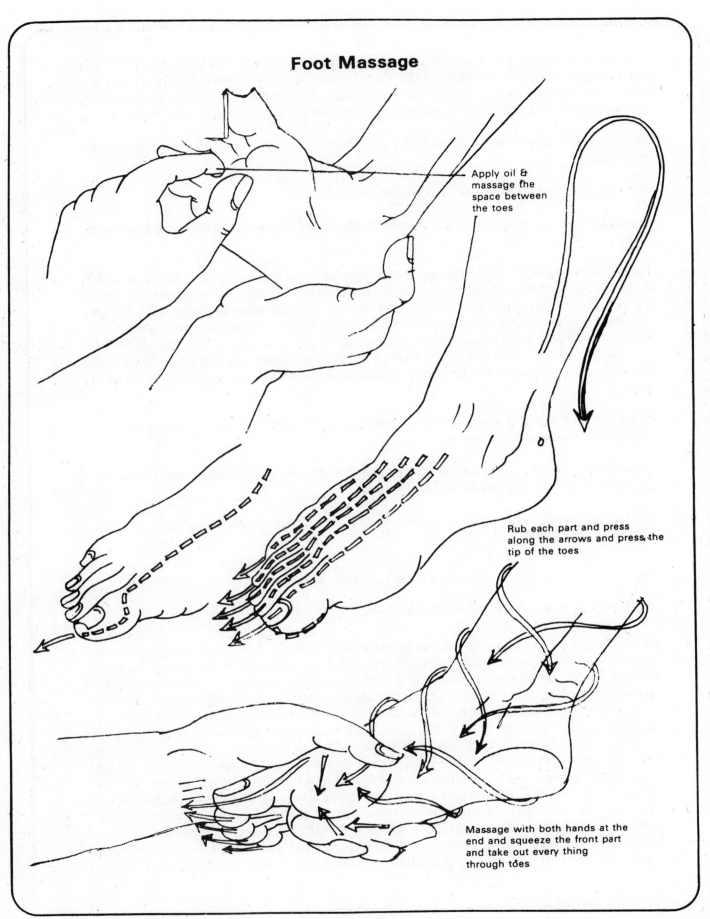

Apply oil & massage the space between the toes

Rub each part and press along the arrows and press the tip of the toes

Massage with both hands at the end and squeeze the front part and take out every thing through toes from ankles to toes. Block the circulation on one side with the hand that holds the foot by the heel—and with the help of the thumb—and fingers of the other hand move—and press on the top—and sole simultaneously along with the bones leading from ankles to the toes. Massage in the space inbetween these bones is very useful.

The massage of the toes starts from the joint . . . where the toe bone joints the footbone.

Give pressure—and circular movement to each joint.

Twist the toes . . . couple of times on either side—and massage the area in between the toes.

Put oil on the nails . . . and massage the in between area with your fingers—preferably make a claw-like shape with your palms—and put your fingers in between the toes of the person getting massage. Rub simultaneously with all your fingers—Pull the toes . . . Hold the toe with your thumb—and forefinger. Start from the joint of the toe—press—and bring your hand which is pressing—and rubbing . . the base of the toe . . . Hold it tightly—and twist it . . . then pull it with pressure—and let your fingers slip through the end part of the toes, applying maximum pressure on the end part of the toes.

Turn the foot around again. Press it forwards and backwards–and then squeeze the whole foot from ankles to toes.

Then start squeezing the whole foot starting from the upper leg doing a crisscross movement with both hands simultaneously.

In the end twist—and pull each toe—and shake off hands after each toe.
Clap . . . and relax . . .

Massage of the Back

Back area is from tail bone to cerebellum.

There are five divisions of the spine where oil should be applied—and circular movement should be made to enhance circulation. Massage of the back is not as much related to the lymphatic system as it is with the nervous system. There is a chain of sympathetic ganglions on either side of the spine—and by massaging this area as shown in the diagrams, the discharge of spinal motoneurons is increased, which helps the weak muscles. Massage here is like slow stretching . . . which provides relaxation to muscles, also there is a direct canal filled with CSF (cerebro-spinal fluid) connecting the base of the spinal column with the core of the brain. According to the ancient system of Tantras, the human organism has seven centres of consciousness specified along the spinal column. In fact a massager is not concerned with the chakras which are the centres of consciousness—or psychic centres but—as he massages the spine and works with the back he manipulates the sympathetic chain of ganglions, the sympathetic—and para-sympathetic nervous system which form the autonomous nervous system in the body. To manipulate these psychic centres without counting the actual number of vertebrae of the spinal column we have found a fantastic device which has a physiological correlation with the chakras.

(1) **Base of the spine**—seat of 1st chakra
(2) End part of the hip bone is in alignment with the 2nd chakra in the spine.
(3) End part of the rib cage is in alignment with the 3rd chakra in the spine.
(4) End part of the shoulder blades is in alignment with the 4th chakra in spine.
(5) End part of the collar-bone joint is in alignment with the 5th chakra in spine.

The massager should locate these points by following straight alignment with the parts mentioned above; oil these areas—and massage them with thumbs in a circular movement.

Two areas in the back are overstressed—and the massager should give special attention to these areas:

(1) Waist region
(2) Shoulder region.

Ask the person getting massage to lie down on his stomach as in the beginning of the massage.

Fix the two thumbs of either hand at the base of the spine—and move hands—as shown in the diagram. The massager should remember that during the whole period of back massage the thumbs will be placed on either side of the vertebral column whereas the hands (with fingers) will work on the whole back area—as shown by the arrows in the diagram of the back massage.

Tapping is done as usual before fixing the thumbs for rubbing—and pressing part of the massage.

Kneading of the waist area—is done after tapping—then shaking is done wherever possible.

Each time the hands are removed—they should be clapped. Clapping charges the hands. Oil should be touched with fingers and applied to the back. For spreading oil the massager should make circular movement, bearable pressure should be applied while rubbing—and the thumbs should remain located on either side of the spine. The person getting massage should place his or her arm in a position where he or she feels relaxed, preferably under the forehead when the lower back is massaged—and alongside of the body when massage is given to the upper back area. Extra kneading—and pressing should be done to the area where the person getting the massage feels pain.

The massager should work with the spine applying oil—and rubbing in the five above mentioned divisions, and gradually move from the base to the top.

The massage of the back ends with a rapid movement made by hands with thumbs fixed on either side of the vertebral columns and then lifting the skin with two fingers on the sides of the vertebral column. The skin of a healthy person lifts up easily—and

Upper Back Massage

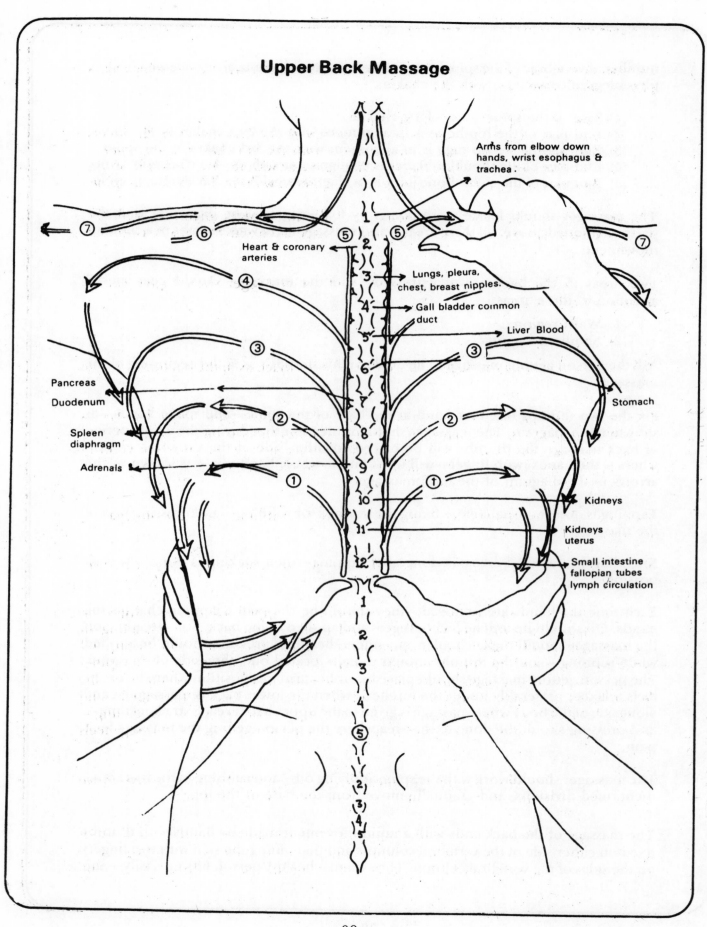

Lower Back Massage

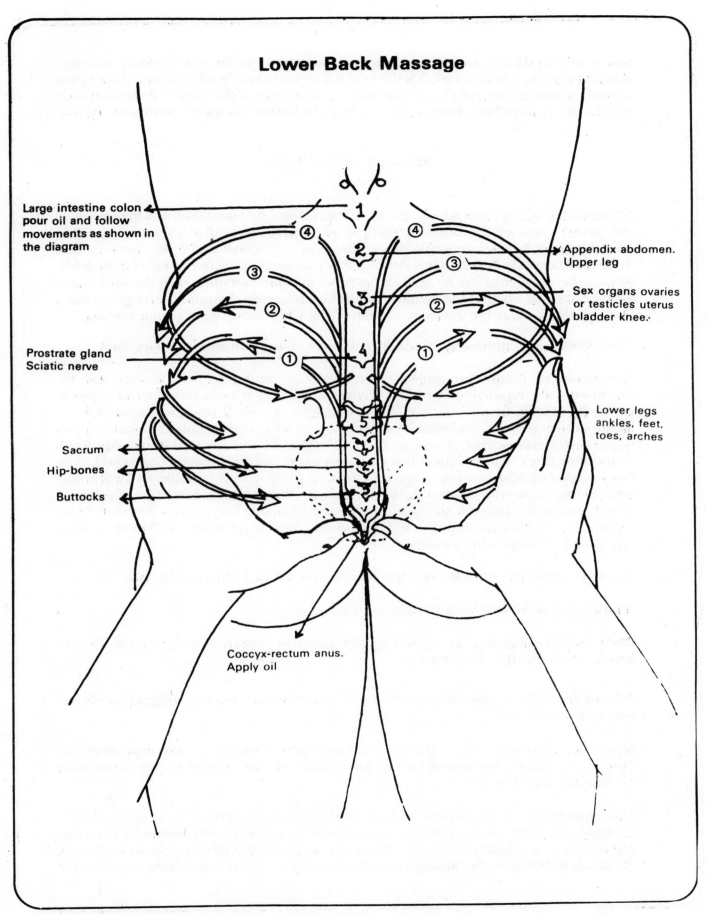

Large intestine colon pour oil and follow movements as shown in the diagram

Appendix abdomen. Upper leg

Sex organs ovaries or testicles uterus bladder knee.

Prostrate gland Sciatic nerve

Lower legs ankles, feet, toes, arches

Sacrum

Hip-bones

Buttocks

Coccyx-rectum anus. Apply oil

wherever the skin is not lifting properly—and seems to be stuck—more massage should be given. This is a sign that the internal organ related with this part of the spine is not functioning properly. Lifting the skin on either side of the spine is done with both hands—and moves from down to up . . . (from the base of the spine to the neck region).

Massage of the Front

The massage of the front part of the torso starts from the navel. Navel is the centre of the preservation of the body. According to Ayurveda—and Yoga both—navel is considered to be an important place. There is a function of 72,000 (seventy two thousand) nerves in this area. It is through this area the child is connected with the body of his or her mother before he or she is born. All vital life fluids flow from the body of the mother into the body of the child through this area, even the pranic energy operates through this area as the external nostrils of the child are clogged—and inactive.

The person getting massage should be asked to lie down on his or her back.

The massager should then put his three fingers excluding the little finger—and the thumb into the depth of the navel to feel the pulsation. The pulsation shall be register-ed by the middle finger—in case of every healthy person. If pulsation is not felt . . . let the subject relax . . . and relax your own fingers, try to feel it again. If no pulsation is registered by either of the three-fingers the subject will be having problems of stomach —and intestines. This is called dislocation of navel (nabhi or naaf). This could have been caused by lifting heavy weights, pulling or pushing heavy articles or by running a lot. In each case some effort to bring the dislocated nerve back in its original position is to be made. Sucking the air through a blower—causing vacuum set the nerve in its right position. This method should be properly learnt from an expert before exercis-ing it on any subject in massage.

Then the messager should pour the oil into the navel, until navel is full.

There is a folk belief about the shape of navel in India.

Deep navel is regarded as a good quality navel.In Indian iconography Gods are always shown with a deep navel.

Protuded navel is supposed to be demonic—and persons having bulging navels are eternally dissatisfied.

The navel is also the centre of gravity in human body. There are many lymph nodes in this area—and circular movement clockwise given by the massager helps circulation of digestive fluids in this area.

The massager should then press on both sides at the place where the rib cage ends. On the right side of the person getting massage is the location of his or her liver and on the left side his or her stomach is located. Pain experienced by the subject on any side during the gentle pressing by the massager indicates problem in that organ. Pain experienced

Front Body Massage

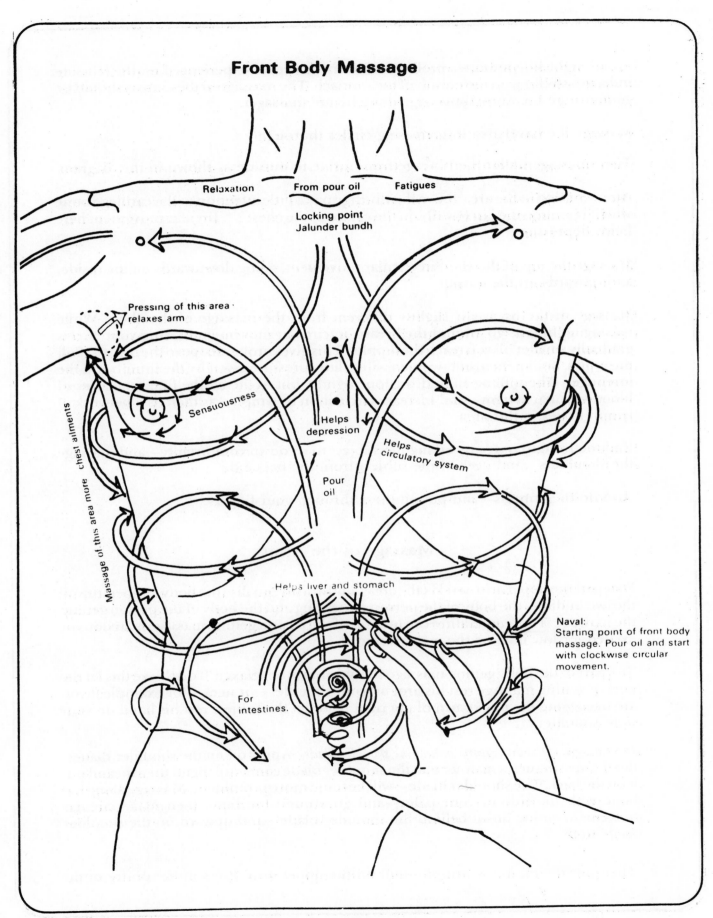

Relaxation
From pour oil
Fatigues

Locking point
Jalunder bundh

Pressing of this area
relaxes arm

Sensuousness

Helps
depression

Helps
circulatory system

Pour
oil

Massage of this area more   chest ailments

Helps liver and stomach

For
intestines.

Naval:
Starting point of front body
massage. Pour oil and start
with clockwise circular
movement.

on the right side indicates problem of liver—and pain experienced on the left side indicates swelling on the mouth of the stomach. The massage in these areas should be gentler than the normal massage done by the massager.

Massage the navel area in increasing circles thoroughly.

Then massage under the rib-cage from inside to outside as shown in the diagram.

After working in the area above the rib-cage pay a little attention to the cartilege bone which is joining the last few ribs in the centre of the chest . . . circular movement here helps depression.

Massage the top of the chest in circular movement, going downwards on the inside, and upwards on the outside.

Massage of the breasts is slightly different from the massage of the chest. While massaging breasts go around the breasts in circular movement making your circles gradually smaller till you reach the nipples. This gives proper shape to the breasts. Pull the nipple both in men and women with a little pressure given by the thumb and the forefinger. The pulling should be done lightly, but excite all the fine capillaries of blood vescular system—and increase circulation of lymph—as there is a network of lymph nodes in this area.

End the front massage by asking the subject to sit down comfortably—and massage the shoulders—and neck of the subject from the back side.

Also do the armpits—and put oil there through your fingers.

Massage of the Arms

First part the upper arm to relax the areas, and also to equalise the body temperature of the two bodies—the body of the person massaging and the body of the person getting the massage. The temperature can increase if the person getting massage is anxious or excited, or low if he or she is depressed.

The part of the body getting massage should always be relaxed. To achieve this let the person getting massage rest his arm on your shoulder—or neck—for example if you are massaging the upper arm of the right hand let the subject rest his hand on your right shoulder.

The massage of the arms starts behind the shoulder blades. Apply oil on the shoulder blades. Put the arm in such a manner that the shoulder blade comes up. Bend the arm and put it on the back. The shoulder blade—will become more prominent. Massage along the bone with the side of your palm—and go around the bone then make circular movement, going down behind the shoulder blade—and upward on the shoulder blade itself.

Then put the oil in the armpit—and on the upper arm. Press in the centre of the

Arm Massage

indicates a circular gentle rubbing movement.

anticlockwise

clockwise

1. Follows the musculature and stop at biseps.

2. Come from back and stop at brachialis.

3. Start from external carpi radialis longus— and come to ext. pollicis brevis.

4. Press Flexor pollicis longus.

5. Press Flexor artinaculum.

①
②
③
④
⑤

Earth
Water
Fire
Intelligence
Grasp
Ambitions
Air
Adoptability · TY
Rub gently
Massage
Massage
Man
Twist them gently
Akash
Determination
Expression
Passions
Sex

These two work in cooperation helping one gain one-pointedness & cure nervousness

These two form a lock which helps centring cures nervousness

Finger tips are related with consciousness their engagement is engagement of consciousness

Arm Massage

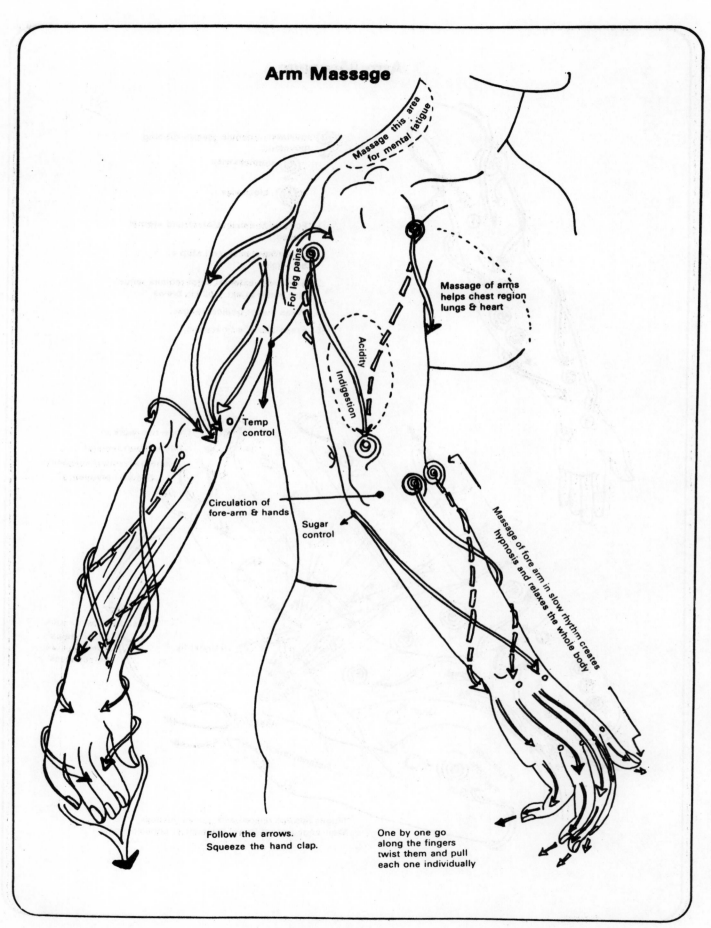

Massage this area for mental fatigue

For leg pains

Massage of arms helps chest region lungs & heart

Acidity

Indigestion

Temp control

Circulation of fore-arm & hands

Sugar control

Massage of fore arm in slow rhythm creates hypnosis and relaxes the whole body

Follow the arrows.
Squeeze the hand clap.

One by one go
along the fingers
twist them and pull
each one individually

armpit until you feel the pulsation, of the carotid artery located in this area. After applying pressure—and feeling the pulsation make circular movement to excite the lymph nodes which are spread around in this area. Do some kneading—pressing—and squeezing on the front size of the armpit.

After kneading the upper arm start rubbing—and pressing of the upper arm following the musculature. See the diagram—and follow the movement shown by arrows. Put your thumb on the outer part of the upper arm, and go down making simultaneously inward—and downward movement towards the inside of the elbow using your hands. Alternate the same practice to cover both sides of the upper arm.

There are important points in the upper arm. They can be located by pressing gently on the sides of the arms where the muscles of the shoulders come to an end. These pressure points are called Marmas in Ayurveda—and according to their definition one experiences severe pain when these points are rightly pressed. Give circular movement on these points—and continue massage of the upper arm.

Then stimulate the lymph nodes situated in the hollow of the elbow. Stimulate it from the other side also, working alternating the fingers on the sides of the bone in elbow and in the hollow of the elbow.

Massage of the lower arm starts with blocking the inside (pink side) by putting one finger in the hollow of the elbow near the tenden and putting the other finger on the side of the bone of the elbow on the reverse side. After blocking the pink side work on the thumb side of the lower arm. Go down along the thumb—and the forefinger. Then reverse the process—and block the other side—and work on the remaining three fingers on the pink side. The blockage will be experienced as numbness on the side which has been blocked.

Then do the kneading of the lower arm, and spread oil.

In rubbing, thumb of the hand goes downwards from inside of the elbow towards the backside of the lower arm.

For massaging the hands first block the pink side, by putting one finger on the middle of the wrist (back side)—and other finger on the pink side of the wrist, after this the massage should be given on the thumb side. The process should be reversed to massage the hand on the pink side.

Then massage the whole arm again.

After this massage the inner part of the hands (the palms) thoroughly specially in the middle region.

Then the massage should be given to the middle part of the palms, where the fingers start.

Put oil in the nails, and massage with all your fingers formed in the shape of a claw all the inbetween spaces between the fingers.

Then massage the wrist and the back side of the hand (turn hands).

Then go down from wrist to each finger, pressing alternately back—and front of the palms—and the fingers. Work at each joint, twist the fingers—and finally pull them—as done in the feet. Shake hands after each finger.

In the end do the whole arm again . . . by rubbing—and squeezing at the same time making a crisscross movement with both of your hands press the palm—and fingers jointly—and pull clap—and end the massage of the hand.

Head Massage

The head is the centre of the whole nervous system and it is the first organ which crystalizes in form in the process of development of the foetus. The head is bigger in size and heaviest in weight (normally it takes three months for a child to balance his head). In childhood, the head has an opening. The top of the cranium is soft over the section of mid-brain. This part can be easily seen and one can see this soft part pulsating. This part is called the *Brahmand in yogic* language and is termed the *Tenth Gate*. The body has ten gates from which *prana* leaves:

> anus
> genitals
> mouth
> two nostrils
> two eyes
> two ears
> *Brahmand*   (the top of the cranium,
>   about 8 fingers width from the eyebrows).

The *Brahmand* opening is meant to provide energy to the child. Within a period of nine months this part of the skull becomes stiff and hard like a bone, then the opening does not exist. Head massage very carefully done, at this age is very nourishing. It is only during this period of nine months that through this soft, porous part of the skull nourishing oils may be supplied and provide the child with more energy with which to think and learn and remember and have better sight for the rest of his life. After these nine months, not much oil can reach the brain. Head massage done during these nine months energises the cerebro-spinal fluid and strengthens the nervous system of the child. This soft spot (*Brahmand*) is supposed to breathe and absorb *prana,* solar radiations and other forms of subtle rays of energy present in the atmosphere. In *yoga,* this place is supposed to be the seat of consciousness, the seat of self and the abode of self in unconscious-conscious state called *Samadhi*. This portion is directly above the pineal body, the olfactory lobe; the section called the mid-brain. This area is in the direct path of the mysterious serpent power (*Kundalini*) which flows through *Shushumna*. Application of nourishing oils to this area helps the brain and nervous system.

Oil applied to the head is absorbed into the roots of the hair, which, in turn, are connected with nerve fibres leading directly to the brain. A picture of the brain is printed at the end of this book to show the two areas in the brain from where the cerebro-spinal fluid circulates inside and outside the brain. These two areas have openings from the inside to the outside of the brain where the network of nerve capillaries is spread.

Oil strengthens the hair and removes dryness which is responsible for the brittle hair and for so many scalp disorders. By relaxing muscles and nerves, fatigue is eliminated from the system.

Head massage is good any time, except for the time after food and conditions under which massage is prohibited. But it is especially good in the morning before bathing and, if necessary, in the evening after having finished work for the day.

Massage of the forehead, or application of pastes such as sandalwood paste, or the application of *malai* or cream from milk calms the system and creates good feelings in the brain, making one feel high. The application of clay cools. Application of sandalwood paste before meditation on the forehead is a common practise in India. It helps one meditate and relax. (*To make sandalwood paste, rub a piece of sandalwood against a stone and add a few drops of water, a pinch of organic camphor and a pinch of saffron. Rub to dissolve the camphor and saffron. Add water as needed.*)

Massage of the temples improves eyesight and creates a centred state of awareness.

Massage of the eyebrows relaxes the whole body and is especially beneficial for the eyes and the nervous system.

Massage of the forehead increases sight and the power of concentration.

Head massage in particular increases the supply of fresh oxygen and glucose to the brain, along with the circulation of the life-giving sap of cerebro-spinal fluid. It increases the growth hormones and enzymes necessary for the growth and development of the brain, it also increases the level of *pranic* energy.

Scalp massage cures dryness, loss of hair and premature baldness.

Head massage should be included in the daily schedule.

Oils to use for Head Massage :

Sesame oil extracted from black sesame seeds is supposed to be the best for hair. Sesame oil alone may be used, or mustard oil alone may be used by males. Coconut oil may be used by females.

There are more oils which are beneficial for head massage.

>Amla oil
>Bhringraj oil
>Brahmi Amla oil
>Brahmi Amla Shikakai
>Brahmi Amla Bhringraj Shikakai

Sesame oil plus Almond oil plus **Sandalwood oil**
Sesame oil plus Almond oil plus **Jasmine oil**
Sesame oil plus Almond oil
Pumpkin seed oil
Kahu oil
Coriander oil
Mixture of *Kahu* plus Pumpkin plus Almond oil.

There are three important spots on the head :

1. First spot is located at 8 fingerwidth of the subject from eyebrows upwards. This is a soft spot at birth—and gets hard with the completion of the ninth month. In India (northern part) a pad with oil (cotton cloth or cotton ball soaked in oil) is put on that spot, after the birth. This is the tenth gate mentioned in yoga scriptures.

2. The second spot is where there is the cowlick. The hairs at this spot are turning in the form of a whorl—sometimes clockwise sometimes anticlockwise. This area is also known as the crest. Hindus grow hairs in this area—and those hairs are specially called by a name . . . SHIKHA . . . This is supposed to be a sign of being a Hindu. They twist these hairs—and knot them together. This practice is essential for those who practice Pranayama.

3. The third spot is where the neck meets the skull, the place of the brain stem, medulla oblongata.

The massager should make the subject sit down in a comfortable position—and then ask the subject to measure the first point—by measuring eight fingerwidth above the eyebrows—put his finger on the spot—and pour oil there. Then the mixing of the oil with both the hands as shown in the diagram is done.

The head massage starts with measuring the spot located at a distance of eight fingerwidths from the eyebrows—and no patting or kneading is done on the head as it is done on the other parts of the body. Here massage starts after pouring the oil. Then the oil is uniformly distributed by the fingers of both the hands of the massager by rubbing from the spot simultaneously towards the sides of the skull upto temples. Then oil is poured at the second spot —and oil is again uniformly distributed by the fingers towards the side—and finally oil is poured on the third spot and the oil is again distributed by the same method of using all the fingers.

Then pressing of the point on the medulla oblongata is done—and the fingers are brought towards the forehead along with the sides of the two ears. See the illustration.

Then pounding of the head with hand joint loosely together is done to excite the fine capillaries of the circulatory system—and the nervous system.

Then the rubbing of the important spots as shown in the illustrations is done, hairs are twisted at the cowlick and the tenth gate.

After this the pressing of the skull with both the hands is done with a little additional pressure.

In the end (before doing the massage of the face and the forehead) the hairs are twisted on all the three spots—and pulled gently.

Then starts the massage of the forehead from the mind. Point of the eyebrows the location of the sixth chakra. The massager should carefully study the illustration—and massage the face.

The head massage ends after doing the face massage.

The massager should rub his fingers gently on the scalp—and pull the hairs on the top of the cranium the location of the seventh chakra—and clap.

If one wants better results with the massage, a drop of oil should be poured into each ear. The subject should move his lower jaws to let the oil go deeper inside the ear. Also a drop of rose water should be dropped into the eyes.

Head Massage

1. Measure eight finger widths.
2. Pour oil.
3. Mix oil with finger tips symmetrically down both sides.

8. Finger widths.

1. Twist hair-lock according to cowlick
2. Pour oil
3. Mix.

92

Head Massage

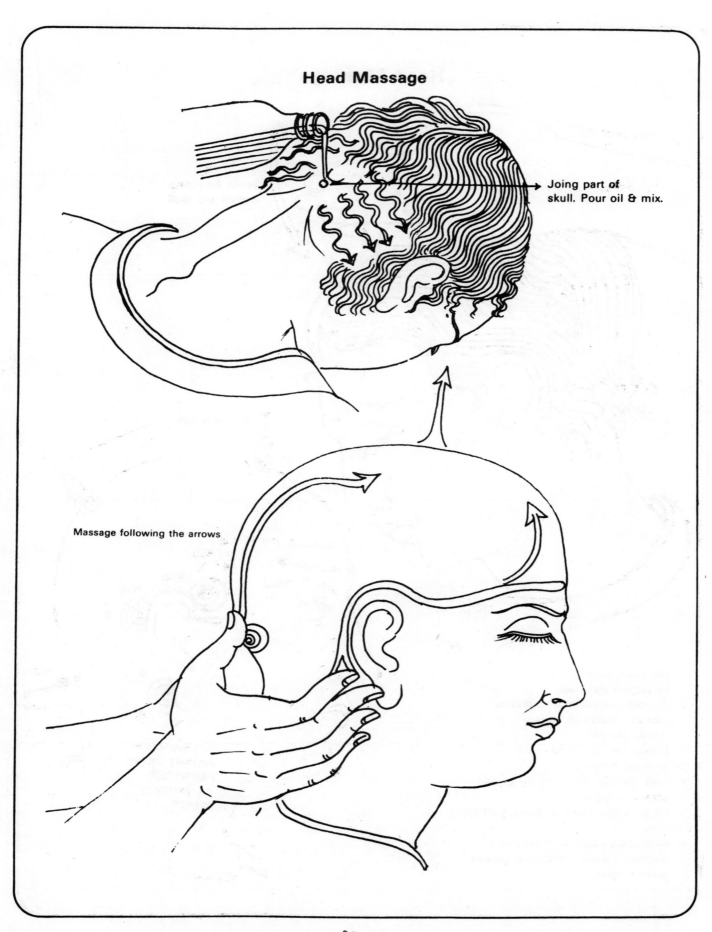

Joing part of skull. Pour oil & mix.

Massage following the arrows

Head Massage

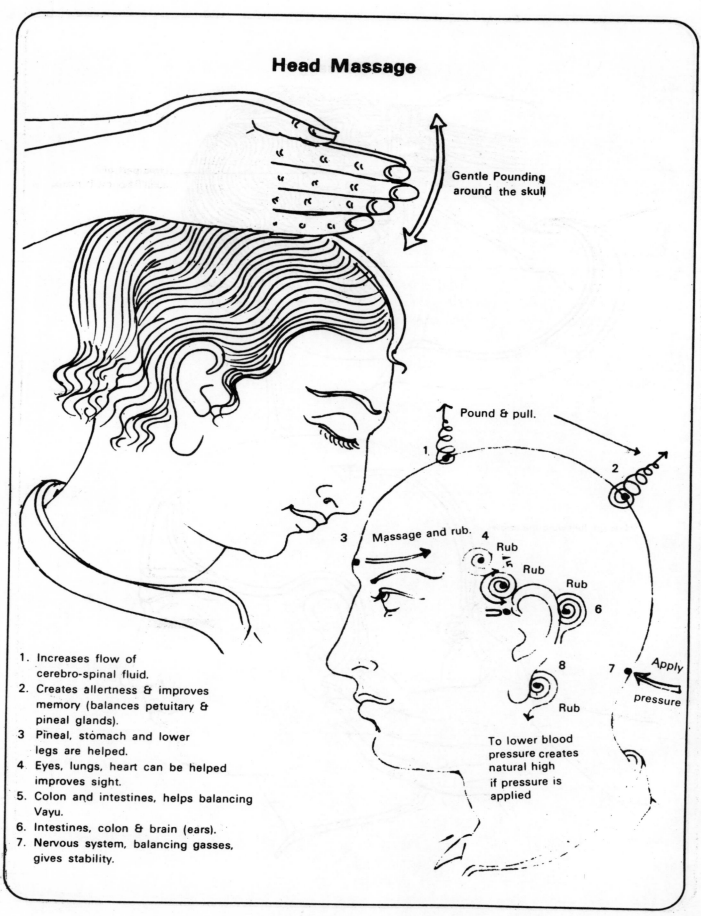

Gentle Pounding around the skull

Pound & pull.

Massage and rub.

Rub

Rub

Rub

Apply pressure

Rub

To lower blood pressure creates natural high if pressure is applied

1. Increases flow of cerebro-spinal fluid.
2. Creates allertness & improves memory (balances petuitary & pineal glands).
3. Pineal, stomach and lower legs are helped.
4. Eyes, lungs, heart can be helped improves sight.
5. Colon and intestines, helps balancing Vayu.
6. Intestines, colon & brain (ears).
7. Nervous system, balancing gasses, gives stability.

Head Massage

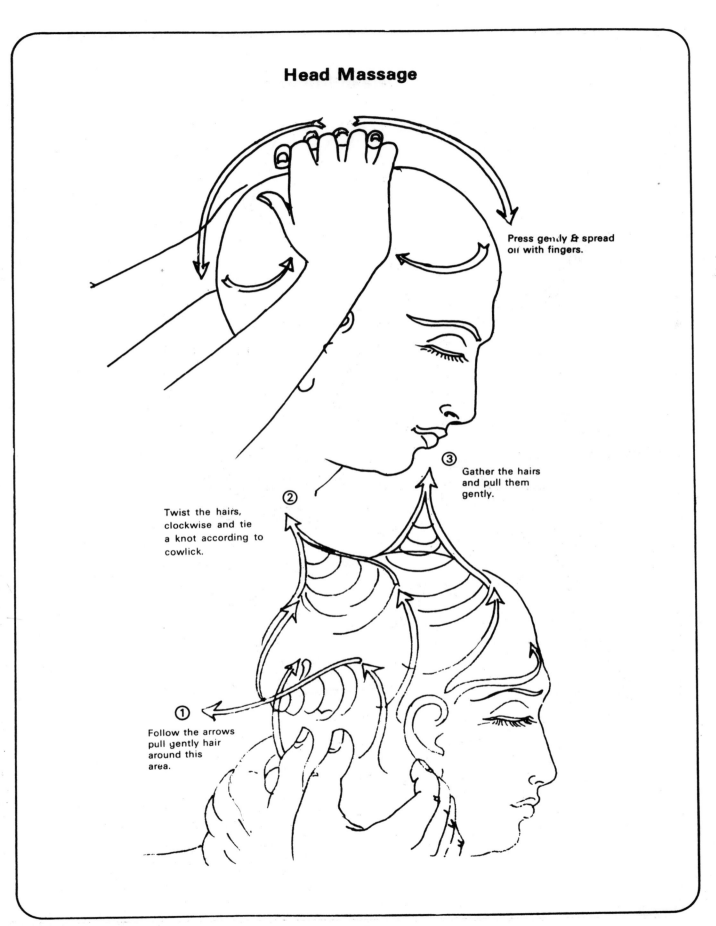

Press gently & spread oil with fingers.

③ Gather the hairs and pull them gently.

Twist the hairs, clockwise and tie a knot according to cowlick.

②

① Follow the arrows pull gently hair around this area.

Head Massage

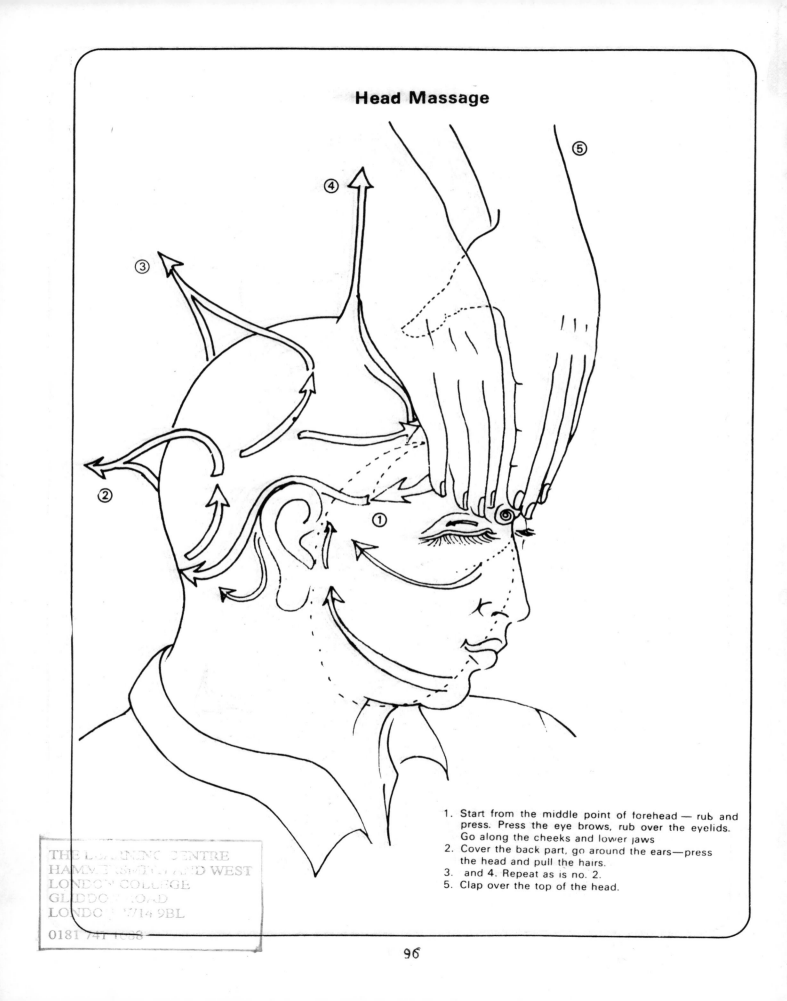

1. Start from the middle point of forehead — rub and press. Press the eye brows, rub over the eyelids. Go along the cheeks and lower jaws
2. Cover the back part, go around the ears—press the head and pull the hairs.
3. and 4. Repeat as is no. 2.
5. Clap over the top of the head.